The Natural

SUPERWOMAN

AVERY

a member of

Penguin Group (USA) Inc.

New York

The Natural
SUPERWOMAN

The Scientifically Backed Program for

Feeling Great, Looking Younger, and

Enjoying Amazing Energy at Any Age

Uzzi Reiss, M.D., OB/GYN,
and *Yfat Reiss Gendell*

Published by the Penguin Group

Penguin Group (USA) Inc., 375 Hudson Street, New York, New York 10014, USA • Penguin Group (Canada), 90 Eglinton Avenue East, Suite 700, Toronto, Ontario M4P 2Y3, Canada (a division of Pearson Canada Inc.) • Penguin Books Ltd, 80 Strand, London WC2R 0RL, England • Penguin Ireland, 25 St Stephen's Green, Dublin 2, Ireland (a division of Penguin Books Ltd) • Penguin Group (Australia), 250 Camberwell Road, Camberwell, Victoria 3124, Australia (a division of Pearson Australia Group Pty Ltd) • Penguin Books India Pvt Ltd, 11 Community Centre, Panchsheel Park, New Delhi– 110 017, India • Penguin Group (NZ), 67 Apollo Drive, Rosedale, North Shore 0632, New Zealand (a division of Pearson New Zealand Ltd) • Penguin Books (South Africa) (Pty) Ltd, 24 Sturdee Avenue, Rosebank, Johannesburg 2196, South Africa

Penguin Books Ltd, Registered Offices: 80 Strand, London WC2R 0RL, England

Most Avery books are available at special quantity discounts for bulk purchase for sales promotions, premiums, fund-raising, and educational needs. Special books or book excerpts also can be created to fit specific needs. For details, write Penguin Group (USA) Inc. Special Markets, 375 Hudson Street, New York, NY 10014.

The Library of Congress catalogued the hardcover as follows:

Reiss, Uzzi.
The natural superwoman : the scientifically backed program for feeling great, looking younger, and enjoying amazing energy at any age / Uzzi Reiss and Yfat Reiss Gendell.
p.   cm.
Includes bibliographical references and index.
ISBN: 978-1-58333-285-6
1. Women—Health and hygiene.   2. Hormone therapy.   3. Menopause—Hormone therapy.
I. Reiss Gendell, Yfat.   II. Title.
RA778.R428   2007   2007032775
613'.04244—dc22

ISBN 978-1-58333-324-2 (paperback edition)

Printed in the United States of America
10 9 8 7 6 5 4 3 2

Book design by Meighan Cavanaugh

To my good friend Richard Fura, a pioneer compounding pharmacist who passed away too soon.

This book could not have been written without the support, love, and invaluable advice of my partner of thirty-five years, Yael Reiss. Many of my initial epiphanies regarding how bioidentical hormones work came from the information she contributed regarding her personal experiences.

—Uzzi Reiss

To my partner in life, Bradley H. Gendell, who provided endless love and support, and who happily took over our wedding-planning duties so that my father and I could write this book, at the long dining table of our loft in chilly New York City and my folks' round kitchen table in sunny Los Angeles.

—Yfat Reiss Gendell

ACKNOWLEDGMENTS

We gratefully acknowledge the help of:

Our highly testosterone-driven agent Peter H. McGuigan, who fought to place this project into the hands of the right editors.

Our editor, Lucia Watson, and our publisher, Megan Newman, at Avery, who expressed enthusiasm for this project from the beginning and gave us the latitude and support to write the book we believe in.

And the millions of women around the world who refused to accept no for an answer and demanded that bioidentical hormones become available to those who choose them. You are the Natural Superwomen for whom this book is written.

AUTHOR'S NOTE

I make some strong statements throughout this book. Some may be unfamiliar to the physicians with whom you speak about your own health-care goals. However contrary the information is to what you or your physicians have heard, each statement is based on scientific studies conducted at established facilities and published in recognized medical journals. Space concerns prevented us from listing more than a very small fraction of these. You can find a complete and constantly updated listing of references on my website, at www.UzziReissMD.com, organized by corresponding chapter and page number. After my previous book, *Natural Hormone Balance for Women*, was published, many readers wrote to let me know that having these references available allowed them to speak to their physicians about implementing the recommendations outlined in the book. I encourage you to print out this detailed listing of references and bring it to the attention of any physician who questions your desire to try any of the programs described in the book.

—Uzzi Reiss

CONTENTS

Introduction:
Do You Feel Like Yourself?

Today, otherwise healthy women are exhausted. They are asked to do more with less, to give more than they have, and to create more than is actually required. Between what's expected of them and what they expect of themselves, the twenty-four hours of each day are simply not enough. And at the end of the day, there's very little available to help them recharge.

Slowing down is not an option for most of us. So what is?

As a gynecologist specializing in optimizing nutrition and hormonal health, I regularly see both stay-at-home moms and women who run media empires, and they describe similar symptoms of exhaustion. No matter how they spend their days, the experiences and feelings women report are the same: their bodies and minds are constantly on overdrive. They are overwhelmed.

It doesn't have to be this way.

MEET THE NATURAL SUPERWOMAN

With more than thirty years' experience in a medical practice focusing on women's health, I believe that by simply paying attention to four basic principles, or four pillars, any woman—no matter how busy she is or how much money she has in her bank account—can arm herself with what she requires to manage the expectations, obligations, and commitments that fill her days and nights. These four pillars include:

the nutrition pillar (proper diet and supplements, where desired)
the activity maintenance pillar (work, exercise, sex, and hobbies)
the hormone balance pillar (*basics*, where required, and *extras*, where desired)
the mind and mood pillar (mental well-being and control)

I believe that by simply fueling their bodies and minds with the principles of these four pillars, women can take control of their own well-being and become the best versions of themselves, by maximizing and exceeding the genetic predisposition they started life with.

This is what being a Natural Superwoman is all about.

In my Beverly Hills, California–based practice, I teach my patients how to focus on these four areas of their lives—diet, hormones, mental well-being, and activity maintenance. These are tools that allow them to become the best version of themselves, allowing them to achieve their goals, while finally having the ability to take a breath and enjoy the real gifts of their lives—their families, jobs, friends, and personal time.

Would you like to become a Natural Superwoman? It can be as simple as tweaking one aspect of your life in each of the four pillars for one week. Try it and see if you begin to feel like a better version of yourself. My bet is that you will.

THE FOUR PILLARS
OF THE NATURAL SUPERWOMAN

Do More with Less

In order to operate at peak performance, any machine, animal, or process must first address the basic requirements for running "glitch free," which means a process runs more *efficiently*, because any process is slowed down or requires repeating in order to correct the mistakes caused by glitches. Running more efficiently means you are able to do more with less. Multinational corporations expend enormous energy and resources to insure their systems and staff members operate with fewer glitches and do more with less. Thinking about your own life and the way you've spent the last seven days, how much time have you devoted to increasing your ability to do more with less?

If your answer is *not much*, don't worry; you've just qualified yourself as a normal busy woman. But if you like the idea of increasing the efficiency of your mind and body and having the ability to do more with less, consider doing what the world's most successful companies do daily—address your mind and body's basic requirements for running glitch free. Natural Superwomen all over the world do this every day, by taking small steps to meet their minds' and bodies' basic requirements, or four pillars.

Your Basic Requirements

The Nutrition Pillar (Proper Diet and Supplements)

This pillar focuses on what and how you eat and how to supplement your nutrition, if you choose to. Among the undesirable symptoms or "glitches" discussed, this pillar offers a special focus on ideal diet for total four pillar maintenance, weight management, and energy level. This pillar also addresses supplements found in fortified foods, and includes an examination of calcium versus magnesium.

The Activity Maintenance Pillar (Work, Exercise, Sex, and Hobbies)

Just as getting into the habit of brushing your teeth helps you maintain good oral hygiene throughout your life, so too does maintaining other habits that engage your mind and body. Your commitment to continuing your professional development, physical activity, sexual expression, and preferred social and leisure activities is imperative to maintaining a sense of youth, energy, memory, focus, and mood, no matter what your age. You'll find a full discussion of the nutrition and activity pillar in Part One.

THE HORMONE BALANCE PILLAR
(*BASICS*, WHERE REQUIRED, AND *EXTRAS*, WHERE DESIRED)

Whether or not you elect to maximize your hormone levels, every Natural Superwoman should be able to identify the major hormone groups and the glitches, or undesirable symptoms, affecting this pillar when hormone levels are not optimized, including those relating to estrogen, progesterone, melatonin, DHEA, pregnenolone, thyroid, testosterone, and human growth hormone. In this section, I address hormone-based contraception and concerns about bioidentical versus chemicalized hormones, and explain what safe options are available to women who choose to use hormone replacement therapy (HRT) or hormone-based contraception (birth control pills) at any age. Finally, I'll give you special information on breast cancer and hormone-based cardiovascular support. You'll find a full discussion of this pillar in Part Two.

THE MIND AND MOOD PILLAR
(MENTAL WELL-BEING AND CONTROL)

Most women understand that managing stress levels is important, but you may not know that you must monitor the way you respond to physical and emotional stress in order to manage all other pillars. This pillar addresses overall stress management, cortisol management, and adrenal deficiency, but also how Natural Superwomen can use all four pillars—positive mood control, nutrition, hormone balance, and activity—to naturally manage depression, anxiety, insomnia, and other challenges to increase overall efficiency and enhance performance. You'll find a full discussion of this pillar in Part Four.

How Your Understanding of the Four Pillars Can Make a Difference

Now that you have a basic idea of what the four pillars are, I'd like to show you how understanding the four pillars can make a difference to your everyday life. Let's say you feel tired. Which of the four pillars require your attention in order to remedy your feeling of fatigue so you can proceed with your day?

Obviously, the answer is all four. You may be tired because of a hormonal deficiency, possibly related to where you are in your menstrual cycle, or if you are no longer menstruating, an insufficiency related to one of several menopausal hormone adjustments (hormone balance pillar), poor diet (nutrition pillar), or your mental state, perhaps because you are depressed (mind and mood pillar), or, finally, you may be tired because you have been inactive lately (activity pillar).

But you really didn't need this book for that answer, did you?

Now let's look at the way you would address this same challenge as a Natural Superwoman. Start with the first pillar mentioned in our answer, the hormone balance pillar. Rather than simply concluding that your fatigue may be related to a menstrual or menopausal condition, you would first determine whether you're meeting the basic requirements needed to avoid fatigue *within* the hormone balance pillar. Specifically, are your adrenal gland function or your estrogen, thyroid, and human growth hormone levels where they should be in order to meet the basic requirements of the hormone balance pillar alone?

Begin with Yourself

Rather than run for a blood test, your first instinct should be to ask yourself some questions. The way a Natural Superwoman *feels* helps her determine what kinds of examinations she requires—your own feelings serve as your best Step One in almost every instance. After all, *you* are the ultimate authority on how your body feels and functions, irrespective of blood tests.

If you are tired, answer the following:

> *How* are you tired? *When* are you tired? Close your eyes and try to identify *how* your fatigue manifests itself.
>
> Are you more tired in the morning, during the day, or in the evening?
>
> If you feel tired in the morning, do you find that you have a hard time getting out of bed when your alarm goes off?
>
> How does your skin feel? Is it dry?
>
> Do you perspire more or less quickly than usual when you exercise? Do you perspire at all?
>
> Do you feel cold in the morning? If so, which parts of you feel that way?
>
> If you feel cold during the day, do you find that you have low energy?
>
> Do you have a short fuse or a hot temper?
>
> Do you have a more pessimistic outlook on things than you normally would?
>
> Do you feel listless and unable to motivate?
>
> In general, do you have less "zing" in your step?
>
> Do you ever feel dizzy when you try to stand?
>
> Do you sometimes find that you can't stand to be around loud noise?
>
> If you feel fatigued in the evening, do you find that this discourages you from socializing?
>
> Do you feel like this every day, or just some days?
>
> Are you ever so tired that you can't fall asleep properly?
>
> Is your sleep not restful, making you feel even more fatigued the following day?

Okay, take a deep breath. We're done with the questions.

When a patient first comes to me and shares that she feels fatigued, these are the questions I ask. Ideally, the two of us use her answers to address her symptoms and concerns and then she's on her way. That's the *first* time. The next time she feels any of the symptoms we discussed, she asks *herself* these questions and together we address her basic requirements more quickly. Her own ability to communicate how she feels helps me determine what I should test for. But *she's* the one who knows what's going on in her body and is the ultimate authority on whether or not she feels better.

After a while, paying attention to how you feel becomes second nature. In the same way you learn what happens physically when you are hungry—rumbling tummy, headache, low energy, or mild irritability—knowing what types of physical signs are associated with insufficiencies in your hormone balance pillar allows you to identify and address them more quickly. And once you know the symptoms, meeting your own needs, solving glitches, and becoming a more efficient version of you becomes second nature, too.

Using Your Understanding of Symptoms Like a Natural Superwoman

So what do all those questions reveal? Some didn't even seem to relate to fatigue, right? In fact, the answer to each question points to a different hormone balance pillar insufficiency, every one of which could lead to fatigue. Pinpointing which one ails you makes all the difference in addressing what is actually going on in your body and helping you and your doctor resolve your glitch more quickly and completely.

For example, if you feel tired in the morning and are slow to "get going," if your hands and feet feel cold, if you have dry skin and low or no perspiration when you are physically active, then your fatigue is likely caused by a lower than ideal thyroid hormone level.

On the other hand, if you feel both physical and emotional exhaustion throughout the day—perhaps you become dizzy when you try to stand or loud noise is unbearable to you—your fatigue is likely caused by a less than ideal function level of your adrenal gland.

If you feel listless throughout the day and must force yourself to participate in physical activity, *particularly* in the days before your menstrual period begins (if you are menstruating), then your fatigue is likely caused by a less than ideal level of your estrogen hormone. Because estrogen levels naturally dive to low levels in the days before your menstrual period, a girl or woman with a generally less than ideal estrogen level suffers far more fatigue than the average woman or girl.

And finally, if your fatigue is accompanied by general social disinterest, a lack of confidence, a feeling of hopelessness, and a general lack of appreciation for life's unexpected "zings," then your fatigue may be caused by a less than ideal level of human growth hormone, a hormone responsible as much for mental "growth" and development as it is for our height.

Four Pillars Crossovers

The example of fatigue illustrates that the cause of a glitch or condition causing you to be less efficient may involve more than one pillar. As you learn more about each pillar in the coming chapters, conditions that cross over between pillars will be addressed anew as needed. For example, in the case of fatigue, a condition that can result from glitches in all four pillars, options for addressing this condition will be discussed using the principles of each pillar in the corresponding chapter.

Less Than Ideal Is Not Ideal

In the examples above I describe a low hormone or low function level as "less than ideal" because, more often than not, you may feel these unpleasant symptoms long before your blood levels would read abnormal in a blood test. Imagine, here you are, living with fatigue, day after day, enjoying your life less, and your blood levels are normal. How could that be?

Simple. Medicine focuses on keeping you alive. If you are not in jeopardy of dying imminently, then you are "normal." The fact that you are at a point within the range of normal that is less than ideal for you, that is causing you to live less efficiently, is not the primary concern of medicine.

However, when you approach medicine with an understanding of how you feel and how your personal assessment relates to your body's basic needs for nutrition, activity, and hormone balance, you are in a position to elect for care beyond that which is required to keep you alive—you can elect to take steps to improve, become more efficient, and do more with less. And that's the way normal, exhausted women become Natural Superwomen.

ELECTING TO BE A NATURAL SUPERWOMAN AT ANY AGE

While most women become more aware of the basic requirements of their minds and bodies later in life, the fact is that women can elect to use their understanding of the four pillars to maximize their performance at any age.

In many cases, if you are functioning at a less than ideal level in one of your four key areas, chances are, that's the way it's been throughout your life. Many symptoms go untreated until they build and a larger system malfunction develops. At this time, you may discover all sorts of untreated symptoms or glitches. But why wait? Why not address the glitch and become more efficient at any age? Maximizing your four pillars—nutrition, hormones, mind and mood, and activity—can be beneficial at any phase of your life. Though different phases require special attention. For example:

Very Young Women (Age Seventeen and Under)

Young Natural Superwomen may be able to better manage premenstrual and menstrual discomfort, mood swings, and childhood obesity made more severe by hormones commonly found in conventionally grown foods, by chemicals in storage containers, and by other daily environmental hazards.

Women in Their Reproductive Years
(Ages Eighteen to Forty)

During a time when they must balance education, career-building, child care, and relationship maintenance, Natural Superwomen must maximize energy, memory, focus, patience, sexual drive, weight maintenance, and mental well-being. Note that many women will start their reproductive years later than age eighteen and continue this phase long after age forty.

Women in Their Balancing Years
(Ages Forty-One to Fifty-Seven)

Women in this phase are still working in or out of the home *and* raising their children, while often required to begin also caring for aging parents—they act as the bridge between two other generations. In addition to all of the glitches or symptoms of their reproductive years, Natural Superwomen in this age range must be especially vigilant in maintaining all four pillars, as this phase lays the foundation for how successfully they will function in their next phase.

The Freedom and Choices Phase
(Age Fifty-Eight and Up)

While medicine is happy to replace knees, hips, and heart valves in the event that they cannot keep up with the lifestyles of the women who carry them, somehow the less welcomed consequences of menopause are regarded as a "necessary evil" of this life phase. Who says? Natural Superwomen make decisions about what is right for their lifestyles based on what feels right to *them*. During this time, thorough understanding and maintenance of all four pillars can make the difference between living and *living*.

Throughout this book, when a glitch, symptom, or condition I discuss is connected with a particular phase of life, I will address the special challenges of that phase. It is my hope that you will be able to share these lessons in this book with your mother and also with your daughter.

I congratulate you on taking your first step to becoming a Natural Superwoman. By simply taking a few moments to read this and learn that you have options for living without the small annoyances—or even larger, seemingly hopeless challenges—you are beginning an adventure that will allow you to become the person you have always believed you could be.

It's all up to you. Why waste another moment being anything other than the Superwoman version of yourself?

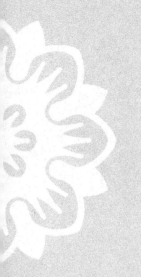

Part One

The Natural Superwoman Lifestyle

1 • Diet and Nutrition: Eating Smart to Achieve Your Ideal Weight

I am blessed every day to meet with women who come from all walks of life and from all over the world. But if there is one single challenge that most women face, it is the quest to lose weight. Here are the common problems that I hear:

"I cannot lose those last four pounds."
"I'm gaining weight around my middle, even though I never have before."
"I'm starving myself and I cannot lose weight."
"I'm eating so healthy and exercising, how can it be that I cannot drop the pounds I want to lose?"

If you find yourself frustrated by similar concerns, you are in good company. Ironically, people in developed nations may arm themselves with a wealth of knowledge about calories, protein, fat, and carbs; commit themselves to more diet regimens; consume more low-fat foods; and produce more best sellers on how to lose weight, but they continue to produce the fattest people on the planet. How can this be?

Some of it can be explained by our attitudes about food consumption itself. If you are unhappy with the way your body has changed over time, or you feel that you cannot meet your weight-loss goals, consider the following questions to determine why, and what you may need to tweak in order to look and feel the way that you desire.

QUICK QUIZ

Today Versus Yesterday

How many calories do you consume every day? More than 1,000? More than 1,500? Two thousand?

Have you gained more than fifteen pounds since high school? More than thirty? Forty-five?

If so, do you consume more calories per day now than you did then?

If you have children, do you weigh ten pounds more than you did before having your first child? More than twenty? More than thirty?

If so, do you consume more calories per day now than before you had a child?

Have you gained more than five pounds in the last year? More than ten? Fifteen?

If so, do you consume more calories per day now than you did a year ago?

Do you gain more than five pounds in the month of December? If so, how many more calories per day do you consume during this time? Is this more than usual?

Sugar Sensitivity

What percentage of your daily calories comes from cereal, bread, pasta, rice, potatoes, and other forms of carbohydrates? More than half?

Are you more likely to eat these foods at breakfast, at lunch, at dinner, or as snacks?

What percentage of your daily calories comes from fruits, fruit juices, desserts, and other sweets? More than half?

Are you more likely to eat these sweet foods at breakfast, in the late afternoon at work, or at night after dinner?

How many glasses of wine or other alcoholic beverages do you enjoy every week? More than four?

When are you more likely to drink wine: on the weekdays, or weekends?

Do you gain your weight evenly around your body, or in your breast or middle section (abdomen, tush, thighs)?

Hormonal Factors

Do you gain more than five pounds in the last week of your cycle? Do you find that you crave more sweets and savory carbohydrates (breads, pasta, etc.) during this time? Do you find you retain water?

If you have experienced a change in your hormone function related to perimenopause or menopause, has your weight increased in conjunction with these changes?

If you take birth control pills, now or ever, have you gained more than five pounds since beginning the pill? More than ten pounds? More than fifteen pounds?

(continued)

Your Weight-Loss Efforts

Do you find that it is harder for you to lose weight today than it was fifteen years ago?

When you diet, do you change *what* you eat, *how much* you eat, or *when* you eat? Or all three?

Do you lose weight if you happen to miss or skip a meal or a snack?

When you diet, do you increase your level of physical activity?

What types of physical activity have historically helped you lose weight? Walking or other light cardio? Running or other more strenuous cardio? Tennis or other vigorous sports? Weight training?

If your answers to the questions posed above reflect that your overall consumption of calories has increased in the last twenty years, if you find that sweets, alcohol, and unfavorable savory carbohydrates affect you more than they used to, or if hormone changes have affected your weight, then making small changes to the way you eat, and how you eat can make a big difference in helping you achieve your weight-loss goals.

THE IDEAL NATURAL SUPERWOMAN DIET

What is the ideal diet? It is one where you maintain your weight and do not accumulate fat in the center of your body, without losing muscle mass and energy level. This diet should also prevent inflammation, the gateway to diabetes, high blood pressure, high cholesterol, arthritis, colitis, osteoporosis, arterial sclerosis, Alzheimer's disease, cancer, and the myriad of other conditions associated with getting older.

The foods that make up this diet must be whole foods, preferably organically grown. Ingredients should not be complicated or contain preservatives, as these products require our bodies to divert energy from maintaining and healing in order to process them. Ideal foods do not contain destructive hydrogenated or partially hydrogenated oils. When possible, eat food that is grown locally and seasonally, as consistently eating the same foods throughout the year may cause you to develop an intolerance or allergy. Additionally, choose fresh foods that appeal to your senses—your eyes and nose—to insure high quality and the full range of vitamins, minerals, and nutrients.

Finally, eat only when actually hungry. Simply feeling hungry may not be a reason to eat. Often, hunger is a symptom of something else. You may be thirsty. You may need to take a walk, or relax and stretch in order to clear your nervous mind. You may not need to eat a full meal; a small snack may suffice.

Natural Superwoman Eating for Weight Maintenance and Quality Life Extension

If my dietary guidelines sound familiar, they should. Eating whole foods is not a unique recommendation, nor should it be. In fact, you may already eat this way. Many of my patients already do, but despite this, some are unable to fully meet their weight management goals. Why?

In certain cases, it is simply because in our world of plenty we have lost perspective on the food portions required to achieve weight loss. Instead, we focus on new diet technologies—advancements in our understanding of the way our bodies process fat, sweet and savory carbohydrates, and salt; our blood types; sleeping patterns, stress levels, and other factors. All of these are important additions to maintaining health and assisting in getting each of us to our weight-loss goals, but none is enough in the long run. Ultimately, only managing your caloric intake, to varying degrees at different ages and health conditions, can get you to the weight you have in mind, and allow you to maintain it. You probably know this already. What you may not know is that there is also a *direct* connection between your management of your caloric intake, at any weight, and your ability to extend your life *and* prevent and fight illness and disease at any age.

Choose a Diet, Any Diet

In a major recent Stanford University study reported in the *Journal of the American Medical Association*, the progress of women on the Zone, Atkins, Ornish, and LEARN diets was compared over one year. The study found that overall, every one of these diets produced *some* weight loss (three to ten pounds), but that even the most effective (ten-pound loss) didn't make very much difference to a woman's overall weight. Ultimately, *only* reducing your caloric intake can help you meet your weight-loss goals.

My philosophy is that as long as you choose whole foods as the underlying nutrient source, the weight management program you choose is less important than how you execute your eating. Different diet principles work for different women—many with diametrically opposed eating guidelines. For example, many women find that they lose weight on a low-carbohydrate diet. Yet 10 percent of the population can eat bread and pasta without gaining weight. Alternatively, a diet containing no animal protein may help many cut fat, but may not provide enough amino acids for other women.

In general, the majority of popular diet programs are most helpful to very overweight men and women. The problem is, irrespective of the diet philosophy women prefer, it seems that most hit a plateau at some point, and are never able to lose the last five to thirty-five pounds they would like, and if they do, they aren't able to keep this weight off.

The Natural Superwoman eating method I will describe here is not a short-term weight-loss diet. In terms of whether you favor high or low carbohydrate intake, vegetarianism or meat-eating, my suggestions are not meant to replace your favorite diet-book program. My feeling is that to the extent you are committed to a particular weight-loss program or eating philosophy, you are free to maintain it, as long as you modify the *amount* you eat in a way that allows you to enjoy the weight loss and health benefits I describe. Of course, as a physician who focuses on nutritional medicine, I also encourage you to seek out whole food sources in anything you eat.

So, what's the difference between your eating and weight-loss program and the one described in this book? Natural Superwoman eating is the only consistently scientifically backed program for meeting your weight-management goals and actively promoting your longevity. It is a lifelong method for getting to your ideal weight, keeping it off, and supporting your body and brain in a manner consistent with quality life extension. Quality life extension is not just living longer; it's living longer while enjoying the physical and mental function that make those extra years worthwhile.

Those Last Pounds

For many women, the only way to lose the last five to thirty-five pounds is to eat less. Interestingly, it is also the case that the only consistently scientifically supported program to extend life span is to eat less. Medical studies have supported this notion for more than seventy years, with consistent results across all the animal species that have been tested, including a thirty-year study on nonhuman primates. The results of these studies have been reproduced hundreds of times.

This method of eating is called "caloric restriction diet." As a physician devoted to promoting ways to extend life, I'm amazed by what an unappetizing name was chosen for a program that represents one of the most exciting developments in the area of diet and nutrition. When most people hear this name, they believe that they are being asked to sign up for torture. For this reason, I call this a caloric *reduction* program. For the average woman seeking to lose those last five to thirty-five pounds, the reduction of caloric intake involved in this eating method is relatively modest and pays amazing dividends, including:

- **Cardiovascular, metabolic, and weight loss.** Caloric reduction improves insulin sensitivity and decreases midsection fat. Caloric reduction also reduces low-density lipoprotein (LDL) cholesterol, triglycerides, and overall weight.

- **Inflammation reduction.** Caloric reduction significantly lowers the rate of mitochondrial free-radical formation in the cells and lowers the markers of oxidative stress. These two mechanisms are the first steps to cell destruction and aging throughout your body. This slows the aging process. Additionally, calorie reduction decreases destructive inflammation factors such as tumor necrosis factor-alpha (TNF alpha) and increases important natural antioxidants such as uric acid.

- **Breast cancer prevention.** As long as you still consume enough calories to meet your nutritional needs, caloric reduction decreases the overall formation of cancer. *Severe* calorie reduction prior to the age of forty decreases the incidence of breast cancer by 53 percent and similar caloric reduction after one pregnancy decreases the incidence of breast cancer by 76 percent.

- **DNA protection.** Calorie reduction protects the genome from damage by increasing DNA repair capacity and decreasing DNA mutation. This slows and can even reverse the aging process.

- **Brain support.** Caloric reduction protects the brain in a number of key ways:

  - Produces new neurons, increases apatosis, or cell maintenance, and preserves the ability of DNA to repair itself in the brain.
  - Decreases brain inflammation, which is the source of degenerative diseases.
  - Decreases oxidative stress (OS), damage caused by free radicals, in the brain.
  - Decreases the toxic effects on your brain and increases memory consolidation.

One study has found that a 50 percent calorie reduction by obese women improves word recall, and another indicated that caloric reduction programs show promise in reducing the incidence of Alzheimer's disease. To put it simply: If you were to ask a genie to overhaul your brain, she would turn back the clock on your cognitive function by crossing her arms and providing you with all of the same benefits that simply reducing your caloric intake does.

- **Bone support.** Although calorie reduction alone may induce bone loss, women experience none if the calorie reduction program is accompanied by physical activity.

- **Muscle support.** Calorie reduction prevents muscle fiber loss and overall muscle mass loss, and preserves the aerobic function of aging muscle. The ability of the body to maintain all of these functions significantly declines with age, but when you engage in calorie reduction, you preserve this ability to maintain muscle. The reason for this is likely because those who engage in calorie reduction do not lose hormone function at the same rate as those who do not reduce caloric intake.

- **Skin support.** Calorie reduction allows many women with significant skin diseases, including eczema, to enjoy significant improvement.

- **Sexual response and function.** Women with anorexia nervosa, a severe, unhealthy extreme of calorie restriction, lose their sexual response and function altogether. On the other hand, the responsible, moderate calorie reduction I describe later in this chapter does not reduce sexual response and function. Moreover, in my clinical experience, women trading in their size 10 jeans for a size 8 enjoy a significant increase in their sexual response and function.

- **Pregnancy benefits.** Pregnant women are often erroneously told to "eat for two," and encouraged to consume as their pregnancy cravings dictate. This often results in a dramatic rise in caloric—particularly empty caloric—consumption and overall weight gain, which can have devastating health consequences for you and your newborn, including an increased incidence of breast cancer.

In my obstetric practice, I recommend an optimal health diet with moderate caloric reduction to obese pregnant patients, who then progress in their healthy pregnancies without gaining weight—effectively losing fat as they gain healthy tissue to be used by their babies—and emerge from these pregnancies weighing less than before their pregnancies. For example, one patient I worked with was seventy-five pounds overweight, weighing 225 pounds. During her pregnancy, she ate healthy foods but reduced the total calories she consumed. As a consequence, her overall weight did not significantly increase throughout the pregnancy, and seventy-two hours after she delivered a healthy child (and placental tissue), she weighed two hundred pounds, having done little more than maintain a calorie reduction eating plan.

In fact, long-term studies indicate that a 30 percent caloric reduction program maintains female reproductive hormones and menstrual cycles, and thus does not compromise women's reproductive health.

- **Thyroid support.** Calorie reduction decreases levels of T_3—the active thyroid hormone. This natural reduction in thyroid hormone function is positive, because it conserves energy and reduces free radicals—two processes associated with longevity. On the other hand, in healthy, lean adult females, inappropriate calorie reduction reduces their T_3 levels and causes them to feel cold. For this reason, when an underweight, fatigued woman visits my office and reports that she feels cold and wishes she had more energy, I often tell her that she does not need thyroid supplements, what she needs is food.

- **Human growth hormone (HGH) support.** HGH provides many benefits beyond simply helping you grow in childhood. Sufficient

HGH levels help you moderate fat accumulation and maintain muscle and skin tone, and provide many other benefits associated with looking and feeling your best. For this reason, anything you can do to maintain or increase your HGH levels is helpful to your overall health. HGH increases during fasting. The reason is to stimulate protein synthesis and prevent protein breakdown, which encourages the body to survive by consuming fat stores, rather than breaking down muscle. In studies on overweight young women with low levels of HGH, simply dieting—not fasting—was shown to produce the same benefits: their HGH levels increased by 60 percent. Logically, the hypothesis follows that calorie reduction through dieting—not fasting—also increases HGH levels.

- **Melatonin support.** As we age, our melatonin level declines. In a twelve-year study using a 30 percent calorie reduction program, age-related melatonin decline was arrested. Melatonin is our human clock. If calorie reduction is able to stop this timepiece from ticking forward, who says we cannot find a mechanism for reversing the direction of its movement?

- **DHEA support.** DHEA preserves your adrenal function and provides numerous benefits outlined in Chapter 7. Long-term calorie reduction slows the age-associated reduction of DHEA levels.

- **Appetite benefits.** Calorie reduction increases adiponectin, a hormone that protects us from cardiovascular disease, cancer, and diabetes, while also decreasing fat. Obese people tend to have larger appetites not just because they're used to eating greater quantities; these people are actually responding to the biochemical effects of their consumption volume. Similarly, when relatively lean persons claim to be satisfied by a lower food volume, they're not kidding around; they're also responding to the biochemical effects of their consumption volume.

- **Other organ support.**

    - **Kidneys.** Caloric reduction mitigates kidney lesions.
    - **Liver.** Obesity increases liver size and the amount of liver fat. Six weeks of calorie reduction decreases liver size by 40 percent, a significant marker for good health.
    - **Eyes.** Calorie reduction significantly improves retina health and slows down its deterioration, slows cataract development, and delays the onset of glaucoma.

    More information from nonhuman primate studies. Ongoing, thirty-year studies on primates suggest that the effect of calorie reduction is universal across species, including humans. Why is information on primates significant to a Natural Superwoman? Studies on primates provide insight into what occurs in humans under similar conditions. In the case of this study, the information on food choices and portions over thirty years could never be collected from human subjects.

- **Disease prevention.** In a human study conducted in a geriatric living facility, sixty residents consumed 2,300 calories per day, as desired. Another set of sixty residents reduced their calories intake to 900 calories only every other day, but made no changes to food quality. In a three-year follow-up, the group that reduced their caloric intake every other day enjoyed a 50 percent decrease in death, a 40 percent decrease in days spent in the hospital, and many other health benefits, including improvement of diabetic condition, asthma, less cold and flu, fewer bladder infections, a decrease in chronic sinusitis, a lower incidence of cardiac arrhythmia, autoimmune disorder, and menopausal-related hot flashes.

What Natural Superwoman wouldn't want to enjoy all of these benefits, in addition to meeting her weight-management goals?

What Is "Caloric Reduction"?

When I introduce my patients to the idea of calorie reduction, their first response is always, "Starving yourself can't be healthy." I'm always glad when they say that, because it gives me the opportunity to remind them that consuming empty calories is also unhealthy. I explain that for most women caloric reduction does not necessarily mean eating dramatically less food, it simply means that you choose foods with a high nutritional value and a lower caloric value.

How much of a reduction in caloric consumption is required to lose weight? The answer is highly individual. Although each of us burns calories at a different rate based on our natural metabolism and activity level, in general most women maintain weight by consuming 1,000 to 1,800 calories a day and lose weight by cutting consumption to 800 to 1,600 calories per day. The amount of calorie reduction required to lose weight is something that you will discover when you take the time to understand what you are consuming today, in order to establish a starting point for reducing consumption.

In my practice, when I encourage patients to list what they eat on a daily basis and add up the caloric value, nine out of ten realize that though they eat a salad for lunch, a relatively light dinner, a fruit snack, and maybe a blended coffee drink, they are inadvertently consuming more calories than they thought. While this does not cause them to gain weight, it certainly won't allow them to lose much.

Here's an example of two lunches that illustrate what I mean:

LUNCH 1
Grilled Steak Caesar Salad with Dressing

1 cup sliced, grilled skirt steak (6 oz.)	360 calories
3 cups romaine lettuce	30 calories
½ cup seasoned croutons	341 calories

3 tablespoons Caesar dressing	234 calories

Total food volume	**4.5 cups of food (plus dressing)**
Total calories	**965 calories**

LUNCH 2
Roasted Turkey Caesar Salad with Reduced-Fat Dressing (no Croutons)

3 cups romaine lettuce	30 calories
1 cup diced lean turkey (6 oz.)	220 calories
3 tablespoons reduced-fat	
Caesar dressing	125 calories

Total food volume	**4.5 cups of food (plus dressing)**
Total calories	**375 calories**

Although many of us have seen this type of illustration before, I find that it often helps to see the numbers again in order to have them sink in. Lunch 1 looks healthy enough—salad with protein and just a couple of croutons (most of which you'll put on the side, but then you think, Mmm, they're yummy so I'll just eat one . . . okay, two . . .). And sure there is dressing on the salad, but you ordered it "light dressing, please," so the chef used only three tablespoons, rather than the usual six tablespoons of dressing. Problem is, the caloric value of this relatively small lunch eats up two-thirds or more of a day's worth of caloric allowance for many women. And that's just lunch!

Certainly, steak is delicious, but so is turkey (or chicken, for that matter), and it saves you 140 calories. And of course, full-fat Caesar dressing and croutons taste better than the reduced-fat stuff and no croutons, but do they taste 450 calories better? By simply making these simple substitutions, you are able to meet your weight-loss goals, or just eat more. For another 100 calories, you could add another four cups of delicious, nutrient- and fiber-filled vegetables:

1 cup sliced mushrooms	15 calories
1 cup diced green pepper	30 calories
1 cup diced celery	15 calories
1 cup diced tomatoes	40 calories

Congratulations, you've just eaten twice the amount of food, while reducing your caloric intake by about 50 percent. Do you feel deprived? Do you feel severely restricted? If your answer is no, I'm happy to hear it, because the calorie reduction program that helps my patients reach and maintain their preferred optimal weight only requires you to reduce your caloric intake by 25 percent—and that's only until you reach your preferred optimal weight.

In the sections that follow, we'll discuss other methods of meeting your caloric consumption goals that also promote health and protect against disease. Now for some specifics.

How to Eat Like a Natural Superwoman

Ask any woman whether she believes she is healthy and she will likely give you a longer explanation, rather than a simple yes or no answer. Ask a woman what her preferred optimal weight is, and she will easily be able to recall a simple three-digit number. Every woman knows what weight makes her feel comfortable, whether it's because her clothes fit better or because this weight allows her to feel comfortable wearing a bathing suit.

What is your preferred optimal weight? Regardless of your current eating philosophy—whether you subscribe to a vegetarian, high-animal-protein, high-whole-grain, or any other diet and eating program—you can lose your last five to thirty pounds by modifying the way you eat your preferred foods, as follows:

- **If you believe that you are not at your preferred optimal weight** (and you are not currently *underweight*), **simply reduce your caloric intake by 25 percent.** You may do this by replacing some portion of your meals with lower-calorie components, or by simply leaving behind one-quarter of every component on your plate. My patients often tell me this is easier to do if you physically remove the excess food from your plate (personally, I require the removal of this portion from the table altogether). Like the idea of food replacement, the notion of leaving behind a portion of your plate (or giving it away, or offering generous-size "tastings" to tablemates) is not new. Country-western singer Dolly Parton referred to this as her "half-diet." It wasn't that she was on half a diet, it's that her diet was to simply eat what she wanted, but just eat half of it.

- **If you lose weight for a while, but then find that your weight loss plateaus** before you have reached your preferred optimal weight (and you are not underweight), **reduce your caloric consumption by another 25 percent.** Be creative in how you cut your calories. Challenge yourself. In the sidebar that follows I share how I enjoy bigger meals, while meeting caloric goals.

- **Once you reach your preferred optimal weight, you can add back half of your most recent cut.** This is the amount of food you should be eating in order to maintain your weight until your body tells you otherwise.

- **Any time you find that you have gained five or more pounds, cut your consumption by 25 percent.** Again, after you return to your preferred optimal weight, you may add back half of that 25 percent. In this way, you'll be able to modulate any changes in the caloric level required by your body.

Eating More Food
While Reducing Overall Calories

To feel satisfied while cutting calories, I suggest that you replace low-volume, high-calorie food with low-calorie, high-volume food. For example, just one cup of cooked brown, long-grain rice contains 215 calories. The same cup of kale or other leafy green vegetable, such as shredded cabbage, contains only 34 calories. That means you can enjoy four cups of kale or shredded cabbage and still decrease your caloric intake by 25 percent, in addition to enjoying the benefits of a vitamin-rich food. That's a lot more food than the one cup of brown rice, and it includes a healthy amount of fiber to make you feel full.

BUT ISN'T BROWN RICE HEALTHFUL?

While brown rice is a more healthful alternative to white rice and other processed grains, its caloric value—and that of any healthy food—is still necessary to consider when your goal is calorie reduction to achieve weight loss. Just because something is good for you, or is organic, or is a delicacy, or is vitamin-packed does not mean that its caloric value is not important. In the example above, brown rice is substituted for another whole food—kale or another leafy green vegetable—that is lower in calories and also good for you.

Another area ideal for decreasing caloric consumption without decreasing the amount of food you eat is your choice of protein sources. For example, a six-ounce piece of top sirloin beef contains 316 to 360 calories, depending on how it is cooked. By contrast, *seven* ounces of roasted turkey breast or shrimp boiled in herb broth contain approximately 200 to 240 calories. That means that you can eat more turkey or shrimp and still reduce your caloric intake by 25 percent.

Making these small choice changes will allow you to continue to eat the same amount of food, but nonetheless enjoy the health and weight maintenance benefits of Natural Superwoman eating.

My Story

Most of the patients I speak to report that losing weight is their number one priority—more than sleeping better, having more energy, improving mood, or increasing sexual response. Sure they want these other things, but if these benefits were to be accompanied by weight *gain*, then they would refuse my recommendations. Why would they put their goal of weight loss before any other goals? These women are not anorexic, nor are they "crazy." They are like you. They are like me.

I am five feet three at the time of this writing (although I hope to grow), and I will be in my sixty-third year (God willing) when this book is published. I think about my diet and weight options on a daily basis, more than every other issue in my life. I exercise at least one to one and a half hours on weekdays and two hours on Saturday and Sunday. My hormones are perfect, and the majority are as they were when I was eighteen because I supplement them. In my specific case, I have learned that I must eat only 800 to 1,000 calories of protein and nonstarchy vegetables a day in order to lose weight. If I eat more, I maintain my weight or gain. With all my exercise, with all my hormone supplements. Remember, this is for *me*, not for you.

It's ironic: I know exactly what it takes for me to lose weight. I know exactly what I will weigh every morning, knowing what and how much I ate and how much I exercised the day before. Still, this goal of losing the last ten pounds (which are like the last fifty pounds or hundred pounds as far as I'm concerned) will only be met when I fully commit to:

Refusing that last glass of wonderful wine.
Passing on a wonderful homemade treat prepared by someone
    I love.
Declining a less desirable food choice or a second helping when I
    am not really hungry, even if that food is vitamin rich, organic,
    green-grass fed, or whole grain, and therefore better for me
    than something that is not.

The Weekend Carnivore

One of the tools I use is choosing lower-calorie protein sources. Because I love steak, I choose to replace the protein source I eat for my weekday dinners with a vegetarian choice. I replace my fish, chicken, or beef during the week with seitan or tofu, both vegetarian food sources from Asia, now found in most supermarkets and natural food stores. This is not because I have strong feelings about vegetarian living, although I have respect for those who choose the lifestyle. I prefer to be a weekday vegan and weekend carnivore because doing so helps me meet my caloric consumption goals.

Six ounces of the average seitan product contains about 180 calories. The average tofu product contains about 150 calories—that's less than half the caloric impact of the steak I eat on the weekends. This simple change in my diet has allowed me to meet my weight-loss goals.

Snacking Between or Before Meals

There will be times when you feel hungry even if you have recently had a well-balanced meal. Alternatively, there will be times when you want to eat before your meal—such as when you will be meeting others at a restaurant where the menu only features foods that you try to avoid or eat in smaller quantities. For these times, I recommend a snack that will chemically reduce your appetite.

To do this, your snack should suppress your production of ghrelin, the hormone that causes you to feel hungry and increase your overall food intake. Ghrelin also quickly moves food out of your stomach, so that you have the ability to eat more. Eating protein suppresses ghrelin. For this reason, while you may be able to eat seemingly endless amounts of carbohydrates like potato chips and pretzels, there is generally a limit to how much protein you are able to eat in one sitting. Carbohydrates also suppress ghrelin to a lesser degree. Your snack should increase your levels of glucagon-like peptide 1 (GLP-1), the satiety hormone that causes you to feel full by preventing food from exiting your stomach. This ultimately decreases our appetite. Fat and protein increase GLP-1.

I recommend combining the following for a great snack that also triggers a feeling of fullness on a chemical level:

One ounce of lean protein, such as shrimp, turkey breast, or tofu (30 calories or less) to suppress ghrelin and increase GLP–1.

+

Four ounces of cucumber and celery sticks, radishes, and bell pepper ribs (less than 40 calories), carbohydrates that further suppress ghrelin and add a source of dietary fiber.

+

One teaspoon of olive oil (40 calories) in a small dish, seasoned with sea salt and pepper, to be used as a dip or dressing for the protein and vegetables to increase GLP–1 and keep the food you're about to eat in your stomach, causing you to feel satisfied by your snack.

+

Two glasses of water (0 calories), along with the carbohydrates and fiber of the vegetables, to provide a greater sense of fullness.

This low-calorie snack adds up to only 110 calories, while curbing your appetite and helping you make better food choices when you must eat out.

WATER

Most of us do not drink water. We drink juice, soda, and coffee. The problem is, we don't have juice or soda circulating in our body. Our bodies contain water and that's what we are meant to drink. Moreover, soda and juice often contain unneeded calories. If your goal is to reduce your calorie consumption, your first priority ought to be substituting juice and soft drinks with water. Your second priority is to choose your water as mindfully as you choose your food: "Whole" water (as in "whole food") is mineralized with sodium, magnesium, and other minerals essential to good health. We lose these minerals when we exercise and sweat and they must be replaced. Conversely, filtered water and most bottled waters available today have had these valuable nutrients removed along with pollutants. Filtered water is like empty calories—it is less useful to our bodies. But it can also be dangerous.

Irrespective of whether you exercise, if you drink filtered water exclusively, you can develop a mineral deficiency, a major problem in our population. So, unless you have a specific doctor's recommendation for a low-salt diet due to hypertension, I strongly recommend that you drink "whole" mineralized water.

Similarly, overconsuming filtered or "empty" water can dilute the existing minerals in your body, causing severe electrolyte deficiency and even electrical changes in the heart, which may lead to a drop in blood pressure and may even cause death.

The other benefit of mineralized (alkaline) water, is that mineralized water increases the alkalinity of the body, neutralizing body acidity. Body acidity is associated with the promotion of disease.

When choosing water, look for water sources that have a pH of 7.5 or above. If you have a favorite water and the bottle doesn't indicate the pH level, call the company to ask.

Can't stand water? Drink green tea. Green tea made with mineralized water tastes better and has many other antioxidant health benefits.

Drink at least eight glasses a day, preferably before and after your meals, or at the very end of your meals, not while you eat. Drinking during your meal dilutes the digestive enzyme responsible for the sterilization and digestion of your food.

By contrast, drinking two glasses of water *before* you start your meal may cause you to eat less, as will replacing your dessert with two glasses of water, an amount that can also substitute for a snack when you've already had more than your goal of caloric intake for the day.

Women who have a tendency to get up at night to empty their bladders should drink the majority of their daily water by seven p.m.

Educate Your Lips
About Natural Superwoman Eating

When we eat, we nourish our mouths and we also feel that we nourish our souls. Unfortunately, while our brains have developed the ability to distinguish between healthy and unhealthy foods, our lips have not. Lips continue to function the way they did for humans living tens of thousands of years ago. Because historically food was not abundant, often was not tasty, and in some cases could not be found for prolonged periods of time, human lips were "trained" to open and eat as much as possible, as long as food sat before them. This allowed humans to hoard nutrients that would support them until the next time food was available. Today, for those of us who live in a world of plenty, in order to enjoy the calorie reduction benefits of Natural Superwoman eating, we must equip our lips with twenty-first-century software. We must empower our lips to *choose*. And teach our lips that there are short- and long-term consequences to opening up and eating. Before allowing food to pass our lips, we must ask:

"Am I hungry?"
"Is this food healthy?"
"Is it prepared healthfully?"

If your answers to these questions are yes, and you have not consumed your caloric limit, then you may eat. But if the food before you is not whole food, or is prepared with excessive fats and high-calorie ingredients, or you've already eaten all that you should, remind your lips that you are far from starving, and that it is in the best interests of your health and waistline to push the food away and live like a Natural Superwoman. Remember, unless you are currently underweight, if your goal is weight loss, then simply being hungry is not necessarily a reason to eat. You must learn to read your body's signals and know when you truly need food and when you are actually just having a craving.

IDEAL NATURAL SUPERWOMAN
NUTRITIONAL SUPPLEMENTS

Why do Natural Superwomen need supplements? It is possible that some younger Natural Superwomen may not. Those who have spent their lives maximizing nutrient absorption by eating only organic goods, avoiding starchy carbohydrates, and refusing empty calories may get all the supplements they need from their food. But the fact is, most of us don't live this way.

Our environment is another reason why modern men and women benefit from nutritional supplements. Our urban and suburban living surroundings are polluted in many ways, and we require additional protections against these atmospheric toxins—the plastics, leads, and other substances that get into our food and water are implanted in our teeth and otherwise fill our homes and work spaces.

Apart from their taking a broad-spectrum multivitamin, I encourage women to arm themselves with ten other simple supplement categories. Some are found in combination pills, others can be consumed by choosing certain foods more often than we otherwise would. In most cases, I would recommend supplementing these important nutrients in addition to mindfully choosing whole foods that also contain these benefits.

The Top Ten Natural Superwoman Nutritional Supplements

Consult a nutrition-oriented physician to determine your individual requirements for the following.

- **Fast-absorbing magnesium**, such as magnesium glycinate. Magnesium provides the base of most of the body's functions, in general, and cellular and hormonal functions in particular. Good sources of magnesium include low-mercury fish, such as halibut, dry roasted nuts (i.e., almonds and cashews), legumes, such as soybeans and black-eyed peas, and leafy green vegetables, such as spinach. Whole-grain cereals and breads, oatmeal, and unpeeled potatoes all have a high unfavorable carbohydrate count and glycemic index, and therefore may not be the ideal sources.

I recommend taking 400 to 1,000 mg daily with food, beginning with the lower dose and increasing by 100 mg daily. Reduce your dosage if you experience soft stool or diarrhea or if you find that you feel too calm, or even sleepy during times that you otherwise wouldn't be. Note that, like other natural remedies, feeling the benefits of magnesium requires supplementing at your personal maximum for six to eight weeks or more.

- **B complex** (B_5, B_6, and the methylated form of folic acid and B_{12}). This group of nutrients is essential for adrenal function support, and helps convert proteins, fats, and carbohydrates into energy, which is necessary for healthy skin and eyes, and red blood cell production and maintenance, among other essential functions. Good sources of B complex include lean meats and poultry, fish, egg whites, small legumes (such as lentils and soybeans), cabbage, and watermelon.

  I recommend taking 25 to 100 mg of B complex daily, with food. Separately, an ideal dose of B_6 is two to three times the amount of the other B vitamins; methylated form of B_{12}, 1,000 micrograms, twice daily, with food; and methylated form of folic acid, 800 mcg to 2 to 3 mg daily.

- **Fish oil (DHA/EPA).** Fish oil is a major nutritional anti-inflammatory. Adequate levels of DHA/EPA are found in *wild* fish; studies indicate that farmed fish contains only a fraction of DHA/EPA. In order to limit exposure to mercury, choose types of fish that are smaller, and are therefore more likely to contain lower levels of mercury.

  I recommend taking 1,000 to 2,000 mg twice daily, with food.

- **Herbal anti-inflammatories.** Guarding against an imbalance in the process of inflammation in your body, foods include most colorful fruits and vegetables, oily fish, and certain nuts, seeds, and herbs like turmeric.

  In my practice, I recommend a proprietary blend, and encourage you to search out the best-quality versions of the following:

  - Pomegranate extract (100 mg daily).
  - Red wine, grape seed extract, and resveratrol combination (100 mg daily, with food). The product you choose should include the extract, skin, seed, and resveratrol. To supplement the treatment of inflammation or active cancer, consider four to six times this dose.
  - Curcumin (turmeric) (600 mg daily, with food).
  - Green tea extract (125 mg daily, with food).

  In my practice I recommend one supplement, Body Guard, that combines all of these.

- **Vitamin D.** This supplement is key to calcium absorption and serves as a strong anti-inflammatory that helps decrease the incidence of breast, prostate, and skin cancers (melanoma). Conversely, inflammation increases when your body is vitamin D deficient, associated with conditions including arthritis, colitis, and osteoporosis. Vitamin D is automatically absorbed through moderate sun exposure, but today concerns about skin cancer and skin damage make this nutrient delivery form less appealing to many women. Prior to supplementing vitamin D, visit your physician to have your level of 25-hydroxy vitamin D checked using the D3 test. Your level should be between 60 and 80 nanograms/ml, and should not be higher than 100 nanograms/ml.

  You may supplement 1,000 i.u. without medical supervision. If you need more, you may do so only under the supervision of your physician. For people with very low levels: 2,000 to 3,000 i.u. or more daily.

- **Coenzyme Q$_{10}$.** This nutrient is a strong antioxidant and a factor in a chain of events that produces energy in the mitochondria, the energy center of each cell in the body. For this reason, it is essential to the health of all human tissue and organs. Beta blockers (used to regulate cardiac conditions), statin medications (taken to control cholesterol), and antidepressant medication suppress the coenzyme Q$_{10}$ and should be supplemented by women who take these medications.

  I recommend supplementing 100 to 300 mg daily with food. Look for the fast-absorbing version of this supplement. Make sure to choose the efficient absorbing type.

- **R-lipoic acid.** This strong antioxidant provides protection against diabetes neuropathy, a nerve disease that produces a loss of sensation in your extremities, among other symptoms.

  I recommend supplementing 150 mg twice daily, with food. Women who take a dosage of 300 mg daily for neuropathy or other conditions should also supplement biotin.

- **Vitamin K$_2$.** This nutrient is a key cardiovascular protector and bone builder. K$_2$ is naturally produced by bacteria in our intestines and is also found in cruciferous and leafy green vegetables, green tea, turnips, tomatoes, raw parsley, cooked broccoli, and olive, soybean, cottonseed, and canola oils. On the other hand, hydrogenated oils may decrease the absorption of vitamin K.

  I recommend supplementing 75 to 150 mcg daily, with food. Look for K$_2$ identified as MK–7 (menaquinone–7), the most bioavailable and only natural form of K$_2$.

- **N-acetyl cysteine (NAC).** This supplement combines three amino acids and functions as a powerful liver detoxifier. NAC's various amino acid building blocks are found in high-protein foods, including meats and dairy products.

I recommend supplementing 500 to 1,000 mg twice daily, with or without food.

- **Tocotrienol and vitamin E complex (gamma, delta, and alpha E).**
  This full range of vitamin E types provides powerful antioxidants helpful for cancer patients and brain support. The vitamin E family can be found in a variety of food oils, such as olive oil, and also in leafy green vegetables, fish, wheat germ, and some berries.

  I recommend supplementing 400 to 800 i.u. of vitamin E complex (gamma, delta, and alpha) and 100 mg of tocotrienol E daily, with food.

Maximizing your body's access to these important basic nutrients on a daily basis provides you with the ideal basis for fighting disease and managing the many complex processes your body and mind must balance in order for you to feel and function at your best.

A WORD ON CHEATING

We must treat our bodies as we would like to treat our relationships—tenderly. In most relationships betrayal is not tolerated. Either partner can destroy their relationship by cheating. With respect to ideal diet and our bodies, some of us cheat at least once a week—if not once a day. Can you imagine what would happen if you cheated on your relationship that often? If your partner did?

Protect your body as you would protect your relationship. Your body won't tell you that your cheating is hurting it, but you will notice that over the years you will get heavier and more sluggish as insulin resistance makes itself known.

And if you do cheat, make better choices. Choose cheat foods with better, purer, whole ingredients, without artificial colors or trans fats.

And remember: Cheating is never an accident. Nor is it beyond your control. You have the right to make the choice to respect your body as a treasured partner. I encourage you to do so.

2 • Activity: The Importance of Living Vibrantly

This pillar addresses physical activity, but also focuses on making sure that you prioritize other important activities. You may know that exercise is important to your health, but keeping a busy social calendar and spending quality time with loved ones may not be activities that you view as essential. In fact, you may be thinking, how can socializing rank as highly as diet and nutrition, mental health, and hormone balance? And that's exactly the reason I added this pillar. This book is not about merely surviving; it is about living in excellence. It is about being the best you can be, becoming the most successful version of yourself. The self that has a varied array of intellectual and leisurely pursuits—the self that is fully engaged in her life. Your social life, romantic life, and your personal passion must be cared for in the same way that you care for your physical health. Elevating yourself to the next level requires these components.

No matter what other responsibilities you have that are vying for your attention, you deserve to have the time to exercise, to express your sexuality, and to enjoy your friends and your partner. Because estrogen predisposes women to be more generous and nurturing, you may be a woman—like many women—who has put yourself last on your list. Instead, you put your partner, your kids, your work, and even your parents before you. Even if you are childless and single, you probably put your friends' requests first. This is a big mistake. You must demand the time required to take care of your own needs. If you won't do it for yourself, do it for the people you otherwise put first—take care of yourself, because they all depend on you.

If you don't, what kind of example are you setting for your kids? What would you say to them if they put themselves last in this way? And if you have no children, what are you teaching your partner or friends about what is okay for them to impose on you? Would you ever ask the same of them? Probably not.

This section provides specific information on the maintenance of physical and sexual expression.

- **Social maintenance.** Estrogen is a social hormone. The presence of higher levels of estrogen in women causes them to be more verbal, social, and willing to make sacrifices to keep the group together. Conversely, the presence of higher levels of testosterone in men makes them more physically, rather than verbally expressive, and may explain why it seems that men lack the social skills that seem second nature to women. In fact, from a hormonal perspective, they do.

  Because social behavior—at all levels—is so intimately connected to feminine identity, maintaining this basic instinct is imperative at every stage of a woman's life. When women are single, they spend time with girlfriends or in search of their partners. If they don't, they should. Later, if women choose to become mothers, they may focus this energy on the management of their new brood, but eventually, they must turn their attention back to feeding their greater need for outside social interaction, even if to a lesser extent.

  Whenever I see women who have become too isolated after the birth of their children, or because they are in relatively new relationship, or even due to a demanding job, some appear a bit flatter and somewhat down. They are thirsty for social interaction, and may not even realize it. For this reason, when I suggest a night out with their girlfriends, they always report feeling energized.

This is not the case for men. Many men can focus on their work to the exclusion of social obligations, and may even prefer to sit home with their partners as soon as the initial courtship ends. A common complaint of my patients is that their husbands change to be completely antisocial once their relationship has become established. In all but the most social men, to some extent, this tendency is by hormonal design.

On the other hand, understanding and honoring your basic feminine need to socialize is essential to being a Natural Superwoman. Irrespective of your current status—whether you are in the throes of an intense new romance, a demanding job, or you've just had a baby—a dinner out once a week is a must. Even if you don't feel the need to change your current schedule, your essential social self will appreciate it. On the other hand, if you are currently overwhelmed by a newborn, if you feel disconnected from your friends due to work travel, or if you are disappointed by the fact that your partner prefers to spend most evenings or weekends at home, you must affirmatively make some time for yourself and spend time with others. Your mental well-being demands it. If this describes you—even if you believe your schedule will not allow it—I urge you to try it once and see if your mood is lifted.

Alternatively, consider carving out social time in a more structured manner. Schedule a weekly (or even monthly) outing for a book club, a bridge club, a knitting circle, a group cooking class with girlfriends— anything that creates an external, scheduled obligation that must be honored by your partner, your family, and by you—that allows you to acknowledge the estrogen that makes you a Natural Superwoman.

MAINTENANCE OF PHYSICAL ACTIVITY

Physically, we were not meant to wake up each morning, take a few steps to the breakfast table, walk to the car or subway or bus stop, then to our desks, take a quick break to visit the water cooler or coffee machine, another excursion to the lunchroom, and then return home to the couch and bed. Many women don't move their bodies at all, or they move too little. On the other hand, some women move way too much. Most women reading this book fall into either the first or last category—they either rarely exercise or they overexercise. Both can be equally ineffective and may even be destructive to your goal of being a Natural Superwoman.

The Problem of Exercising Too Little

I'm certainly not the first physician to write about the importance of exercise and I won't be the last. You have likely heard that exercise:

- **Promotes longevity.** Even moderately strenuous or a small amount of activity will delay death.
- **Prevents cardiovascular disease.** Cardiovascular exercise and weight training prevent and help slow the progress of arterial sclerosis.
- **Prevents cancer.** Exercise decreases the frequency of the four most common types of cancer that kill: breast cancer, colon cancer, prostate cancer, and lung cancer.

If you're in the group that exercises too little or not at all, I am sure that it is not because you don't know that exercise is good for you. More likely, if you don't exercise it's because you don't care for it, or because you feel that you have many other things competing for that time.

However, I'll show you how by investing in one hour of exercise you can achieve the higher quality of life that you are reading this book to learn about. More specifically, moderate exercise:

- **Prevents the effects of aging.** Exercise improves antioxidant function that decreases inflammation and the effects of aging.
- **Treats depression.** Exercise is significantly helpful to depression and overall mental well-being.
- **Improves memory.** Moderate cardiovascular conditioning and strength training actually improve memory.

Exercise also provides energy, better sleep, not to mention all of the aesthetic benefits.

What other one-hour investment helps you look younger, feel better about yourself and your surroundings, and improves your memory? And, in terms of day-to-day benefits, exercise helps you avoid sickness, recover faster, and manage your hectic life more effectively and efficiently. For all of these reasons, even moderate exercise plays an important role in becoming a Natural Superwoman.

What kind of exercise is best? The specific activity is less important than how strenuous it is. Ideally, the exercise you choose should be vigorous enough to make you feel that you are benefiting your body, but not so vigorous that you "overdo it" and feel too tired after your session or too physically uncomfortable to repeat the routine two days later. Burnout goes against the very idea of maintenance.

I challenge you to think of a time when you were physically able to exercise, but decided not to because you were upset, depressed, or just didn't feel like being active. If you ended up going anyway, didn't you feel better once you'd finished? I'm hard-pressed to find a woman who says she did not.

The Problem with Exercising Too Much

As important as it is to exercise, it is just as important not to overdo it. Exercise and strenuous physical activity, especially as we age, increase the amount of oxygen introduced into the muscles and cause intracellular events that can lead to an increase in the formation of free radicals and inflammation. Aging also increases the risk of general muscle injury and the inflammatory response can subject aging muscle to even more oxidative stress.

What is oxidative stress? Although free radicals are naturally produced and can have a positive effect on the immune system, they also have a negative effect on this system by oxidizing protein and DNA. To limit this harmful effect, our body has a complex protection system—our antioxidants. An imbalance between free-radical production and antioxidant defense leads to oxidative stress (OS), which may be involved in the aging process, and the development of diseases like cancer and neurodegenerative diseases like Alzheimer's.

Although it can also be protective, this imbalance of free radicals is sometimes referred to as inflammation.

Exercise can have a positive or a negative effect on oxidative stress, depending on your training load, training type, and your overall ability to engage in the type and amount of activity you've taken on.

Just as people who don't exercise at all maintain this lifestyle despite knowing that exercise helps them live longer and avoid disease, those who overexercise do so irrespective of warnings that it may be too much for their bodies. In some cases, telling a woman who overexercises that she is being extreme and causing damage to her body may elicit a feeling of secret pride or denial. The fact is, the mental high caused by exercise is so great, that, like any other high, it causes some women to ignore physical signs indicating that their training may be too strenuous. Signs of overtraining include fatigue to the point of needing to nap; continuing, excessive pain; and flu-like symptoms.

The problem with this behavior is twofold:

First, overworking your body is similar to overworking a machine—it's no problem if you plan to discard it in the short term, but a terrible idea if you wish to keep using the machine for many years to come. Overexercising is unkind to a maturing body, and doing so undermines quality life extension goals.

Second, inconsistent exercising at high levels—because you want to take that more challenging class, or you want to compete with a workout partner—rather than easing yourself in, significantly stresses the body.

For example, when I observe people walking out of a strenuous spin class, indeed some look great, while others remind me of patients I've seen who have just emerged from surgery or are in the midst of having a heart attack—they look pale, their faces are drawn, some even appear to be hyperventilating.

It can be difficult to recognize that you are overexercising. Despite my medical degree and all of the knowledge gleaned from years of personal interest in nutritional medicine, it took me until age fifty-seven to personally recognize when I am straining my body by pushing it to do too much.

At some point, the act of pushing ourselves—perfect for when we are young—begins to cause significant wear and tear on some more mature human bodies. This is because your body was designed for the sprint of a short, action-filled life, not the long-term marathon that is living to age seventy and beyond. Earlier in human history, our bodies were not concerned with how pushing ourselves physically would affect our golden years (then defined as the years after age forty) because back then people didn't live long enough to need to consider these years. Today, we aim to live past forty and to continue to enjoy a degree of nearly all of the mental, physical, and aesthetic characteristics of youth. I'm here to tell you that if you want to continue to function well into your seventies, you must be more gentle on your equipment. Sure, some world-class athletes are able to push themselves to win international competitions into their forties, but those people represent genetic extremes, not the norm. The majority of women must find a middle ground between maintaining cardiovascular and strength training and a level and frequency of activity that does not produce oxidative stress.

Research shows that well-nourished, well-trained marathon runners demonstrate signs of moderate oxidative damage after a race, so very challenging exercise can cause damage at any age. And as we get older, we become more prone to oxidative damage and muscle injury in recovery.

How Do You Know if You're Overtraining?

When we are young and healthy, it's difficult to recognize that we are overexercising, as the signs are subtle. But, as we age, the signs become easier to recognize. This is not accidental—it's a more pronounced warning signal from your body that you should throttle back. Don't ignore your body's request for activity modification. Listening to your body will prevent an injury or the development of a more serious condition that may completely prevent exercise, whereas simply responding by moderating will allow your body to continue to exercise at this more moderate level for many years to come. What are the signs that should cause you to slow down your exercise regimen?

- **Pre-workout signals.** When a pilot prepares to fly, she first goes through a detailed list of safety checks—every single time she prepares to fly. When you prepare to go to the gym or head out for a run, ask yourself:

  - How are you feeling? Any sign of cold and flu should cause you to take it easy.
  - Are you hearing any grumbles from old injuries?
  - Did you sleep as much or as well as usual?
  - How is your general energy level? Do you feel as strong as usual?

  If you feel signs of cold and flu, feel aches from old injuries, or haven't slept as well, plan a relatively easier workout. The more often you perform this check, the better you will get at recognizing the way your body communicates a need for you to have a lighter day.

- **Post-workout signals**

  - Feeling more sluggish than usual immediately after your workout, two hours later when your exercise high wears off, or the next morning.

- More muscle fatigue than usual immediately after your workout, two hours later, or the next morning.
- Lower-level function at work or in your daily activities following a tough workout. Physical activity should invigorate you and improve your function at work and other daily activities.
- If you feel that you require a nap in the hours after you exercise, despite the fact that you slept well the night before. This should cause you to follow up with a relatively easier workout.
- Relatively small injuries or pains that would not have disturbed you in the past now disturb you.
- Noting that you are slower to recover from injuries, in general. Or that similar injuries sustained in the past affected you less than they do now.
- More frequent colds and bouts of flu that take longer time to recover.

All of these signs should cause you to plan a relatively easier workout or skip a day to let your body recover.

Giving yourself these lighter days will prevent injury and allow you to continue to work out during a more sensitive week.

To explain how significant this issue is, a recent report evidenced the deleterious effect of exercise on infertility. Among the 2,000 women studied who underwent in vitro fertilization (IVF) treatments, the study found that exercising more than four hours a week in the one to nine years prior to IVF treatment was associated with a 40 percent decreased chance of having a live birth and doubled the incidence of pregnancy loss.

Getting More Out of the Time You Exercise Naturally

In order to exercise effectively, I strongly recommend that you maximize your diet, your mental state, and your hormone balance using the recommendations in the other three pillars. The better your baseline wellness, the more prepared your body will be to tolerate the potential strain of physical activity. The following nutritional supplements can also be helpful in getting more out of the time you work out while minimizing your chance of sustaining injury. Each of the following nutritional supplements assists in making your workout more efficient in the specific ways indicated.

> **Note:** The recommendations that follow are not an endorsement or a promotion of the use of nutritional, herbal, or hormonal supplements for the purpose of developing your body beyond your physiological programming.

- **L-arginine.** When taken before exercise, this supplement can reduce the accumulation of lactic acid in your body. Taking 1,000 to 3,000 mg of L-arginine before exercise, you reduce your potential for sustaining injury.

- **D-ribose.** This substance stimulates adenosine triphosphate (ATP), the cellular key to muscle and cardiac activity that improves cardiac function in healthy and unhealthy hearts. In my experience, taking 2,000 mg before exercise and also at any sign of fatigue after exercise will improve your physical performance. My clinical observation is that the effect of this supplement improves with cumulative longer-term use, as well.

- **L-carnitine.** This supplement can protect you from exercise-induced oxidative stress (OS) and can improve exercise tolerance, benefiting training, competition, and recovery. I recommend this supplement in two forms: the first is a powder to be added to water and consumed while exercising. I suggest using 1 to 6 grams; if you use too much you will feel agitated. I also recommend it in a compound that combines

L-carnitine with D-ribose, where a teaspoon contains 2 grams of each. I suggest taking a teaspoon of this combination before and, if needed, also after exercise.

- **L-glutamine.** This supplement promotes muscle glycogen storage, the buildup of sugar energy reserves. L-glutamine is an important fuel for some immune system cells; this substance decreases with prolonged and strenuous exercise. This may partially explain why we experience a dip in immunity when we push our bodies physically. Supplementing L-glutamine has been found to decrease the incidence of illness in endurance athletes. L-glutamine improves sugar balance when taken before or after exercise. I recommend supplementing 2 to 6 grams of L-glutamine before exercise, depending on how strenuous the activity you plan will be.

Physical activity is as important to us as proper diet, stress reduction, and hormonal balance. I encourage you to incorporate this essential component of good health in proportion to your quality life extension goals as a Natural Superwoman.

MAINTAINING SEXUALITY

In the three decades that I have worked as an obstetrician and gynecologist, nearly every one of my patients has shared their sexual function–related concerns and challenges with me.

Most of my patients are busy women. And the most common problem I hear is that as they become busier and more challenged, the maintenance of their sexual selves is one of the first things that goes out the window. I caution you to consider that the busier you become, denying this part of your personal expression will rob you of the opportunity to enjoy a variety of benefits that you desperately need. In other words, when you are busy and distracted, you need your sexual self more than ever.

Of course, when I speak to women who report that they are too busy, tired, or stressed to have sex, some report that they're too tired or distracted to actually miss it. Of course they are. Many times when you get out of the habit of doing something that is good for you, you lose sight of the immediate, short-term benefits associated with this activity. Again, exercising is a perfect example. Most women report that they feel great after they go to the gym. It allows them to be more productive, more calm, and enjoy overall better health. But if they get out of the habit of getting themselves to the gym, they hardly ever report that they miss the way they felt post-workout. Sexuality is just as important to your overall health, productivity, and stress-management goals, and just as easy to get out of the habit of doing.

And with exercise, there will be mornings or evenings or weeks when you don't *feel* like supporting your sexual self or supporting your partner's needs in this way—you're distracted, you're tired, you're otherwise overwhelmed. But the fact is, making a concerted effort to ensure that you are maintaining the *habit* of your sexuality on a weekly or more frequent basis will ensure that you experience the physical and pleasurable benefits of sex regularly.

But, maintaining your sex life is not only about the physical gratification. It is essential to maintaining your relationship, if you are in one. What is unique about sexuality is, when you don't engage it, you can convert a real, loving romantic relationship into a roommate-type relationship in a relatively short period of time. If you've ever allowed this to happen in one of your romantic relationships, you know exactly what I mean.

When a couple does not maintain the sexual component of their relationship, it ultimately affects their overall dynamic. For this reason, I encourage you to get into the *habit* of supporting both your sexual self *and* the sexual component of your relationship by taking structured steps to incorporate sex into your weekly schedule. However silly this sounds, consider putting sex on your calendar. Assign nights where one of you is charged with initiating sexual communication, and another night is the other partner's turn.

Does this sound too scheduled?

Consider the fact that every single aspect of your life is scheduled—going to work, seeing friends, and even taking time to eat. In some cases, you may not be in the mood to go to work or study, but you follow through and enjoy the benefits of doing so. Somehow, in the case of sexuality, we have an expectation that it will continue to be as urgent and spontaneous as it was in the beginning of our relationship. Something about scheduling sex is insulting. Why? Coming to terms with the fact that even good, loving relationships cannot maintain initial sexual urgency is an essential component of maintaining a monogamous relationship. Otherwise, we would all be changing partners every three to six months when the initial sexual high subsides.

You set aside time to go for a run or visit the gym even if you are tired, stressed, and don't feel like it. Similarly, set aside time to communicate sexually with your partner, irrespective of other distractions, and follow through with this plan, even if you don't feel like it at the appointed time. Just as you may not be in the mood to exercise at the scheduled time but end up feeling great afterward, encouraging yourself to follow through with the intention of being sexual will produce a similar result. I have yet to hear a women say, "That was a bad idea."

Of course, you may not feel aroused at the start of the appointed hour, and neither may your partner. I encourage you to take a few minutes to motivate each other to get into the mental frame necessary to make the most of the time that you have set aside. Many patients report that they are able to unwind by taking a warm bath or having a glass of wine in order to reset their mood after a day of distractions. Once you've relaxed, consider that a long-term partner may nonetheless require additional, individual stimulation. Consider that your relationship is worth it.

This investment may be one of the best things you can do for your relationship, and if you are a mother, investing this time to keep it intact is the wisest thing you can do for your kids.

Of course, there will be times in life when sexual expression is not realistic—when you and/or your partner are ill, have extreme schedule constraints, and other challenges. Aside from these extraordinary exceptions, maintaining your sexual identity is an essential component of Natural Superwoman living.

Using the Four Pillars to Maintain Your Sexual Self

As with other efforts to remedy or maximize your experience, optimizing your diet, nutrition, hormone balance, and mental and physical well-being using the recommendations outlined in all four pillars will better prepare your mind and body for the recommendations found below.

- **Mind, mood, and body image.** I have never observed that thin women at a healthy weight have a better sexual function than those who are not at their optimal weight, to any degree. However, I have seen women who carry excess weight to any degree—whether five pounds or fifty pounds—who suppress their sexuality until they lose this weight. This suppression of sexuality may continue for an extended period of time.

In my practice, I spend a great deal of energy reorienting the way these women think about their weight and body image, Here are some common issues among the women I see:

WOMEN NOT IN A RELATIONSHIP

First, women whose body image is so connected to what their scale reads cannot see themselves in a relationship until they have lost their weight. In many cases, these women suppress their sexuality and actively avoid having a relationship, which is a shame in itself. The irony is that, anecdotally, entering into a relationship and being sexual may ultimately be the reason they finally take more aggressive steps to be more healthy and lose weight.

Secondly, if women do lose weight and allow themselves to enter into a relationship, they do become sexual but often express concerns that their partner chose them because of their dress size rather than because of all of the other reasons that make them wonderful. Much more so than other women, they worry that any weight they put on will cause their partners to lose interest in them. What a shame, that the basic human experience of sexual expression is so wrapped up in—what can be—the difference of just a few pounds.

WOMEN IN A RELATIONSHIP

The majority of women who are in relationships and consider themselves overweight—even those who are obese—nonetheless enjoy a healthy attitude about their sexuality. They understand that excess weight has little or no bearing on sexual function, and share themselves openly with their partners. However, some portion of these women feel so deeply embarrassed by their weight, they are unable to confidently express their sexuality with their own partners. In some cases, "overweight" may be as few as ten pounds, but this lack of confidence devastates their sexuality. Does this sound like you?

Whether you entered the relationship at your current weight or you gained weight since the start of your relationship, I encourage you to remind yourself that your partner entered the relationship voluntarily, and chooses to remain in your partnership every morning. In fact, you may be surprised: chances are, your partner may or may not acknowledge a significant change in the way you look. He may regard more pronounced curves as a feminine trait. Either way, you set the tone. Your partner will respond to your attitudes about your own body. If you focus on insecurities, so will he. On the other hand, if you maintain a confident, playful, fun attitude about your private time together, I assure you that your partner will count himself lucky—regardless of what the scale reads.

- **Hormone balance.** The supplement market is flooded with nutritional and herbal remedies that claim to improve every aspect of your sexuality. I do not address these here, as none of them consistently benefits every woman.

Apart from generally optimizing your overall hormone balance, making specific tweaks to your estrogen and testosterone levels can make a big difference in supporting your sexual response and function.

- **Estrogen.** In the absence of estrogen, a woman cannot enjoy much sexual expression. Estrogen lubricates, maintains the elasticity of vaginal walls, enhances breast and nipple sensitivity and overall sensuality, and gives women many of the characteristics associated with the female body. Studies indicate that men are more attracted to women in the times of their cycle when estrogen levels rise. These rising levels of estrogen are associated with making you happier, more social, and more apt to compromise. I call this stage in a women's cycle "the time of romantic sexuality." All of these predispositions also happen to make you more attractive to your sexual partner on a chemical level.

  Your cyclical rise in estrogen level is obviously, biologically, meant to lead to procreation, but even, women who have taken affirmative steps to end their fertility—by having their tubes tied or the insertion of an intrauterine device (IUD)—nonetheless experience a significant rise in their sexual response and function, reporting that they have more frequent intercourse during the week before they ovulate.

  Any time you experience some decrease in your sexual drive, response, or function, always consider that estrogen deficiency might be involved, *even* if you are told that you are within the normal range of estrogen.

- **Testosterone.** A woman's sexuality is also governed by testosterone, working hand in hand with estrogen. While estrogen can lay claim to romantic sexuality, the sexual response associated with testosterone is more proactive and aggressive. But testosterone isn't just about increasing sexual response and function. In addition, this important hormone empowers women with a sense of confidence that allows otherwise less confident women to speak up and make themselves heard. Testosterone also provides women with the whole range of other physical and mental benefits.

For more information on how testosterone affects your sexuality, including information about how to supplement this essential hormone, see Chapter 9.

Part Two

What Bioidentical Hormones Do for the Natural Superwoman

3 • Fact Versus Fiction on the Risks of Hormones

WHY A SUPERWOMAN MUST UNDERSTAND HER HORMONES

Whether you feel comfortable taking bioidentical hormones or would prefer not to, you can't be a Natural Superwoman without understanding your hormones. Familiarizing yourself with the way various components function is as essential as understanding your finances, your job requirements, and how to communicate with your partner or children.

Most women are aware of the general roles played by estrogen and progesterone, but a woman's body includes countless other hormones working together. Additionally, hormones control much more than a woman's sexual and reproductive activities. As I explain throughout this book, hormones play a powerful role in most biological functions and every aspect of your day—from how well you sleep to how easily you get up, how your skin looks when you look at the mirror in the morning to your energy level throughout the day, how well you can recall and perform the tasks you must complete each day, how you feel about the people you must interact with, how much you eat and drink, and much, much more.

To be a Natural Superwoman you must understand what these hormones are and how they affect everything you do, when they decline in your monthly cycle, and when they decline in your *life* cycle. Without the power of this information, you cannot have a full understanding of how your body works, and therefore, how you can make it work to your advantage.

In this section, I will walk you through the key Natural Superwoman hormones, what they do, and how the four pillars affect their levels, where applicable. I will also address why your own natural hormones and bioidentical hormones are safe, and why you should avoid chemicalized hormones at all costs.

Once you understand how powerfully and safely your hormones can support you and your goals when their levels are optimized, you will understand why I believe that all Natural Superwomen should make the personal decision to supplement their hormones.

WHY A NATURAL SUPERWOMAN SHOULD CONSIDER SUPPLEMENTING HORMONES

Every cell in your body is controlled by your hormone levels. Yet you've also likely been made to feel fearful about your own hormones. Does it make sense that something so essential to your living is lying in wait to end your life? Is there any organ or function in your body that is known to be protective and then suddenly deadly?

In general, conventional medicine is most concerned about the hormones that control imminent life or death. Removing your thyroid gland, adrenal gland, or pancreas, for example, will cause you to stop producing thyroid hormone, cortisol, and insulin, respectively, and will insure that you die in short order, unless you supplement any of these hormones. Traditional medicine is comfortable instructing women to take steps to ensure that they have sufficient quantities of these essential hormones. It doesn't bombard women with warnings about the cancer risks of these life-or-death hormones.

On the other hand, hormones that define a woman's sense of vitality, feeling, memory, mental focus, energy, sexuality, sensuality, curiosity, openness, and all the things that add texture and quality to your everyday life experience are treated as if they aren't important because they are not *life or death*. I couldn't imagine my life without these things, can you?

The aim here is to present you with up-to-date scientifically backed data that prove many of the abilities or characteristics you once had, or wish you'd had no matter your age—energy, memory, sexuality, and balanced mood—are hormone-related and can be recaptured by using bioidentical hormones to your benefit. This chapter will also explain why using bioidentical hormones is safe and healthy. They can put you back on the road of being in control, as opposed to a feeling of being controlled.

In my practice, I see some 6,000 women a year, all of them focused on maintaining their hormonal power. These women are neither foolish nor reckless. They are not experimenting, and they are not risking their lives. And they are not self-involved, vanity-obsessed stereotypes. These women are feeling the power of regaining control of their own hormonal system and, in so doing, their lives. They use this power to recapture who they really are, with the perspective of their full years.

I invite you to consider what it would be like to recapture the parts of yourself that you consider to be the best; that is, aspects of your identity that you may no longer be able to experience. You can begin recapturing that power today.

WHAT ARE BIOIDENTICAL HORMONES?

When I speak about bioidentical hormones, I am referring to an exact replica of what your own body produces. When I mean exact replica, I mean exactly, not almost exactly or mostly exactly. Anytime you change the smallest thing about a hormone, you change what that hormone does, how that hormone does it, and the consequence of that hormone's actions. Our body is a sensitive machine, with countless numbers of functions, all designed to work in concert. Small changes to any part of this biochemical dance result in big changes. The way your hormones are produced and function is no exception.

That is why you hear such horror stories in the media and elsewhere about women suffering through side effects, heart disease, breast cancer, failing memory, and other horrific problems. Anytime science tries to alter or better what the wisdom of women's own bodies produces, catastrophic results ensue.

On the other hand, the most dramatic evidence of the safety and health benefits of bioidentical hormones is pregnancy. The hormonal process of pregnancy is extreme. In pregnancy, hormone levels soar—two forms of estrogen levels go up tenfold. The third form of estrogen goes up a *thousand*fold; progesterone levels increase one hundredfold. Human growth hormone (HGH) increases and the available testosterone increases by 20 percent. I wonder why writers who warn women about the consequences of elevating their hormone levels through hormone replacement therapy do not next invade the offices of obstetricians and the halls of maternity wards to interview women who dare to become pregnant and so dramatically change their hormonal profiles? In fact, though hormone levels rise to extreme levels—above what is available in any hormone replacement product—the risk of breast cancer decreases with each full-term pregnancy and the incidence of cardiovascular disease is no higher among women with more children. In other words, despite having their estrogen and progesterone levels elevated in an intense way, over and over again, women remain free of cancer and cardiovascular disease. In fact, allowing your natural levels to decline is unsafe, and leaves you vulnerable to serious health risks that your hormones protect you from every day.

THE ESTROGEN AND PROGESTERONE CONTROVERSY

If estrogen, progesterone, and other bioidentical hormones are so wonderful, why all the controversy? This section is devoted to separating fact from fiction. I began recommending bioidentical hormomes in 1982 and found that doing so is a safe, effective way to resolve the symptoms of hormone deficiency that bring down the quality of life of the women I treat. For example, in the case of estrogen deficiency, dealing with symptoms like night sweats and sleeplessness, foggy memory, and less-than-ideal mood really made a difference to the daily life experience of my patients. I have also found that bioidentical hormones provide benefits to serious health conditions. To be clear, I was prescribing bioidentical hormones, not the medications that women might get from a physician at the start of menopausal or perimenopausal symptoms.

THE WHI STUDY

In 2002, the conclusions of a study called the Women's Health Initiative (WHI) were published and changed everything. The study sought to test the health consequences of taking medications called Premarin (a chemicalized medication used in place of bioidentical estrogen) and Provera (a chemicalized medication used in place of bioidentical progesterone). The study concluded that the use of both Premarin and Provera is associated with breast cancer and cardiovascular disease—a terrifying report for users of these medications. However, when the conclusions of this study were discussed in the news and elsewhere, the distinction between Premarin and Provera and *bioidentical* estrogen and progesterone was not made. A media frenzy emerged, warning that "estrogen" in general is dangerous.

The result of this serious misrepresentation is that a large percentage of chemical *and* bioidentical hormone users became understandably concerned and stopped their estrogen treatments altogether. What followed was even more tragic: millions of women previously on hormone therapy began living with the unpleasant symptoms of estrogen deficiency. These women were also left vulnerable to the many health risks associated with estrogen and progesterone deficiency, *including* breast cancer and cardiovascular disease. You will read more about the health benefits and protection of estrogen and progesterone in the chapters that follow.

Today, it is clear—and the sections that follow will describe—how and why Premarin and Provera are dangerous to women, and how bioidentical estrogen and progesterone are different. They are safe and in fact protect your health. Bioidentical hormones are the exact replicas of the hormones produced by your body, so they do not produce the unwanted side effects and disease associated with nonbioidentical hormones derived from other species or those with a chemical structure that is not an *exact* copy of what you currently produce. I advocate women's hormonal and overall wellness, and once these new reports of safety emerged, it was my hope that the widespread confusion and associated fear would end. Instead, a new set of misleading facts has emerged.

Proponents of chemical and partially chemicalized medications, including Premarin and Provera, sought to salvage the reputation of these medications by blurring the lines between their products (proven unsafe by the WHI study and others) and bioidentical hormones. In fact, these proponents now oppose the term "bioidentical hormones" altogether, claiming that all hormone-type products are the same—that they are all hormone replacement therapy (HRT).

In addition, these same proponents of Premarin and Provera also sought to discredit the findings of the WHI study that found their products to be unsafe. This campaign brought to light all the ways in which the methodology of the WHI study was flawed. One proponent, Dr. Leon Speroff, professor of obstetrics and gynecology at Oregon Health & Science University, and one of the foremost academic authorities on hormonal replacement, announced:

> The negative impact of the Women's Health Initiative is over, we know that study's limitations, we know that some of the conclusions promoted in the media were not correct, and we know that the risks that have been promoted by Women's Health Initiative are incredibly small and perhaps not real.

Unfortunately, the impact of the WHI is not over, because the confusion caused by the study's report and subsequent media coverage resulted in years of misinformation and fear about what is safe and what is not. And although the safety of bioidentical hormones is now reported accurately more and more often, even today reports sometimes suggest that estrogen in general is to blame for any number of health concerns.

THE BIOIDENTICAL HORMONE REVOLUTION

Luckily, in the gap of time between the announcement of the WHI study findings and the redemption of bioidentical hormones in the press, something amazing happened. Women learned about bioidentical hormones and embraced them. Although, after WHI, outside observers continued to believe that all HRT caused cancer and cardiovascular disease, individual women who had previously enjoyed symptom-free living by replacing their hormones did their homework. They dug into the details of the WHI study and discovered that, indeed, the medications used in this study are not the same as bioidentical hormones, and that bioidentical hormones are safe and essential to women's overall disease protection. And a grassroots revolution emerged. Because a physician's prescription is required to obtain bioidentical hormones from a compound pharmacy, many women demanded that their doctors educate themselves on bioidentical hormones in order to provide them with prescriptions. Suddenly, doctors who had no previous interest in bioidentical hormones were reading up and searching for seminars. These women changed the face of all women's health-care history forever. In responding to their own needs, they did more for promoting the health, safety, and benefits of bioidentical hormones than I could do in many lifetimes.

The following section outlines the simple differences between the chemicalized medications used in the WHI study and bioidentical hormones, and explains why bioidentical estrogen and progesterone are safe and essential to your short- and long-term health.

PREMARIN VERSUS BIOIDENTICAL ESTROGEN

When you hear the term "hormone replacement therapy," the substance being replaced is not the bioidentical estrogen discussed here. HRT uses a medication called Premarin, derived from a variety of estrogen types collected from the urine of pregnant mares. In the equine species there are many varieties of estrogen types, all but one different from estrogen produced by the human female. It's logical that a hormone created for another species would be associated with effects that are different from the effects that would be produced by hormones designed for our species, and indeed, this is true. In order to collect this urine, the horses are kept constantly catheterized in constrained stalls.

- **Premarin increases inflammation.** *Bioidentical estrogen in cream form decreases inflammation.* More specifically, bioidentical estradiol (E2, the most widely researched and most commonly used form of bioidentical estrogen, discussed in Chapter 4) in cream form decreases inflammation and, unlike Premarin, does not increase C-reactive protein (CRP), a general marker for inflammation. Note, as with any supplement, how you take bioidentical estradiol matters. In the case of inflammation, bioidentical estradiol cream does not affect CRP, whereas Premarin and bioidentical estradiol in capsule or pill form increase CRP. Why is this significant? CRP is a general inflammation marker; anything that increases CRP also significantly increases inflammation. The simple fact that estradiol does not increase CRP, while Premarin *does*, evinces the vast difference between estradiol and Premarin.

This is important, as increasing inflammation in older women who are already affected will cause their condition to further deteriorate. One of the first things that I observe when patients are switched from Premarin to bioidentical estrogen is that they report a reduction in joint pain, an indicator of an overall reduction in inflammation. Increasing inflammation aggravates other inflammation-related conditions. For example, Premarin can exacerbate the symptoms of lupus.

- **Premarin increases body fat and decreases lean body mass.** *Bioidentical estradiol decreases body fat* and promotes muscle growth and regeneration. In my practice, most patients who switch from Premarin to bioidentical estrogen report that they lose weight.

- **Premarin increases sex-binding globulin.** *Bioidentical estradiol in cream form only mildly affects sex-binding globulin levels.* When sex-binding globulin increases, it decreases the effective levels of other hormones available to women.

- **Premarin increases cardiovascular events, arterial sclerotic disease, and venous thrombosis (blood clots in veins).** *Bioidentical estradiol protects your cardiovascular system* and does not increase blood clots in cream form. In my clinical experience treating more than 20,000 women with bioidentical estrogen, I have not observed a single cardiovascular event associated with estradiol treatment in cream form.

- **Premarin decreases coenzyme Q_{10} and gamma-tocopherol** (gamma-E). These antioxidants are essential to maintaining the cardiovascular system. In my years of experience with bioidentical estrogen, I have never observed any trend wherein coenzyme Q_{10} and gamma-E decreased in the women who supplement bioidentical estrogen.

- **Premarin increases migraine headaches.** *Bioidentical estradiol is an effective treatment for migraine headaches.* For many Premarin users who suffer from migraines, switching to bioidentical estrogen provides the first taste of relief in years.

- **Premarin increases stress incontinence.** Premarin causes leakage of urine when women cough, sneeze, or laugh. In my clinical experience, *bioidentical estradiol reliably decreases stress incontinence.*

- **Premarin increases dry-eye syndrome.** *Bioidentical estrogen decreases dry-eye syndrome.*

As you can see, the risks involving Premarin are substantial. I encourage you to choose the hormone supplement designed for you and save any Premarin in your medicine cabinet for elderly mares in need of equine HRT.

PROVERA VERSUS BIOIDENTICAL PROGESTERONE

In 1982, in addition to maintaining my private practice, I cofounded a PMS clinic in Los Angeles, which was possibly the first of its kind. Since then I've treated tens of thousands of patients with bioidentical progesterone to resolve unwanted symptoms of premenstrual syndrome and also anxiety, insomnia, cramping, and irregular bleeding. In my current practice, more than half of my active patients use bioidentical progesterone and the benefits are dramatic.

However, outside of the walls of my office for many years, a campaign has been waged to blur the lines for women and their health-care providers between bioidentical progesterone and the chemical progesterone produced in labs. For this reason chemicalized medications were given similar names like Provera, Progestin, Progestative, and Progestogen. Even today, many physicians believe that these chemicalized progesterone products are "better for you," and that taking natural, bioidentical hormones is naïve, primitive, and something only wheat germ–drinking extremists do.

To make clear the difference between chemicalized progesterone and bioidentical progesterone, consider how your body responds differently to each.

- **Provera promotes breast cancer;** *bioidentical progesterone* protects against breast cancer by addresing every aspect of what your body requires in order to guard against breast cancer development. Researchers have found that Provera antagonizes the many complex systems that your body employs to protect you from breast cancer, and in some cases studies have found that Provera *promotes* the mechanisms that cause breast cancer.

- **Provera promotes diabetes;** *Provera increases insulin resistance,* which begins the process leading to diabetes; bioidentical progesterone does not have this effect.

- **Provera promotes significant bone loss;** *biodentical progesterone helps you build bone.*

- **Provera harms the cardiovascular system;** *bioidentical progesterone protects your heart.*

- **Provera decreases sleep quality;** *bioidentical progesterone promotes better quality sleep.*

- **Provera affects the immune system negatively;** *bioidentical progesterone promotes your immune system's health.*

- **Provera harms the brain (Provera is known to induce neuron-degenerative diseases);** *bioidentical progesterone critically protects your neurological system.*

- **Provera affects mood** (Provera promotes negative aggressive feelings, panic response, anxiety, and depression); *bioidentical progesterone calms,* relaxes, and positively balances your mood.

- **Research has shown that Provera increases seizures;** *bioidentical pro-gesterone calms your brain* by increasing GABA and allopregnenolone.

Also, in my clinical observation of women treated with Provera by other physicians, I have noted that Provera increases water retention; bioidentical progesterone decreases water retention.

However, I believe that one must give credit where credit is due: Provera has been found to more effectively decrease hot flashes, as compared to bioidentical progesterone. Having said this, I have yet to find a patient who prefers to partially decrease her hot flashes at the cost of increasing her incidence or risk of breast cancer, heart disease, neural deterioration, bone loss, poor mood, poor sleep, hearing loss, increased allergies, seizures, irritable bowel syndrome, and interstitial cystitis.

Despite dozens of reports illustrating the many dangers of Provera listed above and the scientific community's awareness of the dangers associated with Provera, inexplicably the scientific community has not been as vocal as one might expect about how dangerous this medication is. Instead, new and nonetheless similar medications are developed in the hopes that they will not produce the same dangerous side effects. My fear regarding these medications is that it took the medical community thirty years to discover the dangers of Provera. Must we wait another thirty years to learn the same about each of the many of Provera's successors?

You be the judge. My aim in providing you with information on the dangers of chemicalized medications and the safety and benefits of bioidentical estrogen and progesterone is to arm you with the most current scientific data—strong, irrefutable evidence. Should your doctor or anyone else challenge you, encourage the person to take this information and return to school. People who truly focus on women's wellness will be open to discussion and welcome this resource.

4 • Estrogen: The Essence of a Woman

Are you less social?

Do you secretly prefer not to leave the house?

Do you put less focus on your outward appearance—what you wear on your body and face?

Do you spend less time looking in the mirror than you used to?

Are you more pale than you used to be?

Does your skin ever tingle?

Do you see signs of aging lately—your skin is more dry, and more droopy than before?

Have you lost general motivation to get out there and do?

Do most things seem like a chore to you lately?

Do you find that you're less apt to be as generous as you used to be?

Have you lost some of your enthusiasm for physical activity?

Has your sexual drive diminished?

Have you experienced a decrease in the intensity or frequency of orgasm?

Do you notice less vaginal lubrication than before?

Do you sometimes experience anxious panic?

Are you experiencing adult-onset acne?

Do you have body and joint pain?

If you can answer yes to two or more of these questions during part or all of the month, you may have estrogen deficiency or partial estrogen deficiency.

Melanie's Story

Melanie, twenty-one, a successful entertainment industry personality, visited me and explained that she was on the verge of quitting her long-time television series. She reported feeling depressed, sleeping poorly, and having no sex drive or vaginal lubrication. Indeed, her face looked pale and, upon questioning, she confirmed that her periods come on time but have an extremely light flow. She had previously taken Prozac to lift her mood, but stopped taking it when the medication failed to help, though reported that her mood did usually lift slightly in the second week of her cycle. When I tested Melanie's blood hormone levels, her results were all within normal ranges, although I noted that her estrogen levels were at the very lowest end of this acceptable range. I felt that this explained her generally low mood, her light menstrual flow, and her mood lift in the second week of her cycle.

Melanie and I discussed the rise and fall of estrogen in a woman's cycle, and I recommended that Melanie begin supplementing bioidentical estrogen throughout the month, using less when her body produces more on its own according to its cycle. Melanie returned to my office and reported that her sleep had improved immediately and her face had regained its color within a week. The next month, Melanie reported that her other symptoms had resolved and, most important to her, she had regained her sense of well-being and no longer thought about leaving her work.

ESTROGEN BASICS

Estrogen is the hormone that defines you as a Natural Superwoman. Every powerful aspect of you—that you are bright, successful, in control, giving, caring, social, positive, sensual, and sexual—is directly related to the presence of estrogen in your body. Any treatment program that denies you access to this powerful tool necessarily affects all of the traits listed above.

This section aims to provide you with the most current scientific data on what estrogen does, and why—so long as they are an exact replica of what is in your body—estrogen is safe.

Estrogen appears in your body in three forms:

- Estradiol (E2), which is the most potent form of estrogen.
- Estrone (E1), which is found in equal blood levels to E2, but 85 percent weaker than the E2 sister form.
- Estriol (E3), which is the least utilized form of estrogen, despite its equal importance in many function, including protection against breast cancer. E3 is 99 percent weaker than E2.

These three forms of estrogen work together to control and contribute to the function of the following:

- **Cardiovascular system**—your heart, your arteries, your cholesterol level, and your blood pressure.
- **Weight management**—your ability to lose fat, your cravings and hunger level, how quickly you feel full, and whether you binge-eat.
- **Energy**—your overall energy level, your ability to sleep well, your muscle growth and regeneration.
- **Inflammation prevention**—your antioxidant level and your so-called free-radical load.
- **Brain operation**—your memory, your ability to receive and recall information, your neurotransmitter levels, and your general brain health.
- **Bone support**—your overall bone health, and your ability to prevent osteoporosis.
- **Prevention of depression, anxiety, and panic, and of migraine and headache.**
- **Maintenance of other systems**—your hearing, your resistance to developing stress ulcers.

ESTROGEN'S RISE AND FALL
THROUGHOUT A WOMAN'S LIFE

Puberty-Related Estrogen Rise

Until recently, the puberty-related increase of estrogen responsible for the transition of girls to women historically occurred at age fifteen to seventeen. Today, it is common to see fully developed girls at the age of twelve. Why is this?

1. *Overconsumption of calories and overaccumulation of body fat.* Today's girls eat more and weigh more and accumulate more fat than previous generations. There is a direct correlation between weight and fat gain and the onset of *menarche,* the beginning of menstruation. The exact converse of this is the case of athletes in otherwise perfect health, who cease having a period when their body fat dips below a certain level.

2. *Overly estrogenated dairy products.* The milk girls consume is often derived from cows milked during their pregnancies, which causes it to have far higher levels of estrogen overall. Recent studies have confirmed that today's dairy products have dramatically higher levels of estrogen than is commonly recognized.

3. *Environmental pollutants with an estrogenlike effect.* Many environmental pollutants in our air, water and food products and containers behave like estrogen when absorbed by the human body. This causes girls to enter puberty at a younger age.

4. *Liberal consumption of soy products.* Soy and other plants that are rich in *phytoestrogen,* or plant estrogen, are regularly consumed by girls in the form of soy, plants, and even (unknowingly) in processed foods, all of which cause them to enter puberty at a younger age.

   Physicians who work with hormones question the full implications of this early estrogenation of girls' bodies and whether it is connected to a general erosion of women's hormonal systems later in life. Today, adult women are experiencing an estrogen decline and entering into menopause at earlier and earlier ages than previously observed. It is not unusual to see a thirty-five-year-old woman in full-blown menopause.

Early Estrogen Decline

Women are also entering perimenopause at notably younger ages than ever before. Perimenopause (premenopause) occurs five to ten years prior to the onset of menopause, and is characterized by a decline and fluctuation of ovarian hormone production that causes women to experience many subjective sign of estrogen deficiency. The biological definition of perimenopause is an increase in a hormone called follicle-stimulating hormone (FSH). Generally, FSH stimulates ovarian estrogen production. But as ovarian production of estrogen decreases, FSH is produced in greater quantities in an attempt to restore ovarian estrogen production. Although the average women reaches perimenopause between forty-five and fifty, it is no longer surprising to find women entering perimenopause in their late twenties. Twenty-five years ago I would have never seen such young women undergoing this change; back then, it was surprising to see a forty-year-old woman in perimenopause.

In fact, an unprecedented, significantly earlier onset of decline of estrogen production has been observed over the last ten to fifteen years. In my practice, I also see greater numbers of successively younger women who are not in perimenopause but who show significant signs of estrogen deficiency, meaning they are depressed, have memory loss, a decreased sex drive and vaginal lubrication, a reduced menstrual flow, and other symptoms consistent with this condition. Because the normal range of estrogen is wide, these patients' blood levels are within normal levels, but always at the lowest end of normal. In my experience, when this group is treated with bioidentical estrogen, often all of their symptoms are resolved.

I have observed similar trends in the decline of DHEA, pregnenolone, and human growth hormone. I have not observed a similar decline in levels of progesterone. The bottom line? If you experience any of the symptoms described here but have not taken action because you believe that you are too young to enter menopause or perimenopause—think again. In this strange new world in which we live, where hormone production rises and then falls earlier than ever before, no woman is too young. More importantly, the sooner you identify whether your estrogen level is in fact declining, the sooner you will return to feeling and functioning as you prefer to. Moreover, the sooner you address estrogen decline, the more likely you are to regain your full, predecline hormonal profile.

UNDERSTANDING YOUR MONTHLY ESTROGEN FLUCTUATIONS

Knowing when estrogen levels rise and fall throughout your cycle is as important as knowing when you can expect overall estrogen decline in menopause. When you know when your estrogen level will be lower during the month, the way your body feels is no longer haphazard, you can anticipate what days you will feel energetic, optimistic, sexual, sensual, powerful, or sad. If you choose, you can use this knowledge to help balance your estrogen levels during lower points in the month so that you feel and function at your best.

The first day of your heavy menstrual flow is also the first day of your menstrual cycle. Biologically, on this day your body recognizes that you have not conceived, and it begins to prepare for your opportunity to conceive the following month. Your estrogen is low for the first three to five days of your menstrual cycle. This may cause you to feel less than great, but probably better than you do the final days of the last cycle just before your period, when your estrogen is at its lowest. By the fifth to seventh day of your menstrual cycle, your body reenergizes you in preparation for the next attempt to conceive by incrementally raising your estrogen levels until just before day fourteen of your cycle, when ovulation generally occurs. This gradual rise in your estrogen levels does three things to help you procreate:

- It thickens the lining of the uterus, giving the embryo a place to implant.
- It causes you to feel outgoing, romantic, and sensual so that you can find, attract, and connect with the person whom you will procreate with in this cycle.
- It produces cervical mucus to take hold of sperm in the vagina and lead it through the cervical opening to the waiting egg.

HOW RISING ESTROGEN AFFECTS TESTOSTERONE

When estrogen levels rise in your bloodstream, intracellularly, or within the various cells in your body (not necessarily measured in your bloodstream), testosterone goes down, clearing up your skin and making you less confrontational, less aggressive, and generally making you more forgiving. You'll read more about this in Chapter 9.

The day you ovulate is the most critical moment in the biology of your menstrual cycle, sort of like the "last call" in a pub when the bartender alerts everyone to their final opportunity to get an alcoholic beverage. This is your body's last call regarding the opportunity to fertilize your egg for this month. To increase your chances of conceiving, your body sharply drops your estrogen level for less than a day, in order to increase your level of testosterone to arm you with a more proactive form of sexuality generally associated with the human male. With this extra push in motivation, your body hopes that you will make every effort available to have sex and conceive. Because estrogen is also responsible for great female judgment, I personally believe that this drop in estrogen is also designed to diminish your good judgment so that you may be less choosy than usual. Remember, biology doesn't care about good decisions, it only cares about results. Ideally, after this short drop, estrogen levels begin to gradually rise again. However, as women mature, the ovulation-day estrogen drop can become more significant and last a few days longer.

With estrogen on the rise in the week after ovulation, your body is in high spirits because it believes you are pregnant. Then, on day twenty-one, a week before your period, your body catches on that you have not conceived and estrogen levels begin to decline. The older you are, the sooner after ovulation this decline begins, as early as day fifteen of your cycle. With your estrogen levels low and dropping, you may begin to feel some or all of the symptoms associated with estrogen deficiency in mild or extreme forms. Your estrogen reaches its lowest point of the month around the last day of your cycle, the day before you get your period.

If you sometimes experience insomnia, depression, anxiety, memory loss, and other symptoms of low estrogen levels and your symptoms improve in the second week of your cycle and then get worse just before your period, you may be able to resolve this with bioidentical estrogen treatment. In addition, you can enjoy the many health benefits of optimal estrogen levels discussed in the following subsection.

BENEFITS YOU MISS AND HEALTH PROBLEMS YOU FACE WHEN ESTROGEN LEVELS DROP

Although the three forms of estrogen work together, the following benefits are provided by adequate levels of estradiol (E2).

CARDIOVASCULAR HEALTH

Estrogen is essential to the function, maintenance, and disease prevention of the cardiovascular system. *Low levels of estrogen are associated with the following:*

- Decrease in vascular tone.
- Increase in arterial sclerosis.
- Increase in incidence of heart attack and stroke.
- Increase of 60 percent in aortal calcification.

My concern is that these serious downturns in wellness also affect younger women who suffer from estrogen deficiency, who, because of the change in timing of overall estrogen decline discussed earlier, may often have estrogen levels that are as low or lower than those of women in perimenopause. Moreover, the biological changes described above require nearly fifteen years of development in the estrogen-deficient environment before they are expressed in the active disease form—another reason why all women should be focused on maintaining their natural estrogen levels.

In optimal levels, studies indicate that estradiol (E2) provides the following benefits:

- Prevents thickening of the heart walls that causes heart function to deteriorate.
- Prevents heart failure.
- Prevents arterial plaque formation.
- Protects the injured endothelium, the inner layer of the artery where plaque formation begins.
- Lowers LDL (low-density lipoprotein), the "bad" cholesterol.
- Increases nitric oxide (NO), a substance that opens the coronary arteries.
- Prevents the increase of blood pressure.

Estradiol treatment also decreases fibrinogen, a substance that participates in formation of clots, and decreases homocysteine, an inflammation marker. The lower your homocysteine, the better. And most important, it decreases the thickening of the carotid artery walls in the neck, the main source of blood supply to the brain.

ARTERIAL SCLEROSIS AND THE ESTROGEN "GAP" YEARS

For years women were treated with chemicalized estrogen that negatively affected their cardiovascular systems. When these ill effects were brought to light by the much publicized Women's Health Initiative study, reports failed to distinguish between bioidentical estrogen and the medications used in the WHI study, and the initial reaction was to recommend that women stop taking all hormones, including bioidentical estrogen. Many of you reading this may have been affected by this advice and stopped using estrogen.

Since this time, a better understanding of the source of these negative effects has emerged. Science now understands that Provera was the main cause of the negative effect of HRT on the cardiovascular system. In addition, clinical experience illustrates that, beyond being more safe than Provera, estrogen provides more effective relief for the symptoms of estrogen deficiency than do mood medications such as Prozac, anti-anxiety medications such as Xanax, and sleeping medications such as Ambien.

Now that the safety and benefits of bioidentical hormones is better known, a new trend has emerged wherein women are advised to take "estrogen" on its own. In Chapter 5, on progesterone, I will explain why women should never agree to take estrogen without also supplementing bioidentical progesterone, as the two work in partnership to maximize benefit and balance against negatives.

(continued)

And there is another pressing problem—the consequences of the gap in treatment suffered by those women who were advised to stop all HRT in the wake of the WHI study. In the five years between the WHI study that called for women to stop taking estrogen and the new trend described above, wherein women are advised to supplement estrogen on its own, estrogen-deficient women who were not supplementing hormones under the direction of their physicians, began silently developing cardiovascular deterioration.

Now, in restarting their estrogen treatment, women inadvertently worsen their condition, having unknowingly begun the process of developing arterial sclerosis. A recent study indicates that a coronary artery treated with estradiol *in the presence of any arterial sclerosis* will exacerbate this condition. I am not sharing this information in order to further confuse or frighten you. Avoiding this further deterioration is as easy as adding bioidentical progesterone to your estrogen treatment. Even women who may not know whether they have developed cardiovascular disease can safely take estrogen by adding progesterone to their estrogen supplement program. The final takeaway: never agree to supplement estradiol on its own and you will be safe.

WEIGHT MANAGEMENT

I have recommended bioidentical estrogen to at least 10,000 women for more than twenty-five years. Today, a minimum 50 percent of my current active patients use bioidentical estrogen. When I first suggest this treatment, the most common concern I hear is that women think bioidentical estrogen will cause them to gain weight. In fact, just the opposite is true; women commonly gain weight and fat during estrogen decline and are able to lose weight and fat when they supplement estrogen. In the five years leading up to menopause, when estrogen is decreasing, most women gain five to twenty-five pounds. Research shows that bioidentical estradiol applied to the skin increases adiponectin, a substance that helps women lose fat. And it decreases ghrelin, a hormone that causes cravings and generally increases hunger. Interestingly, estrogen decline in women leads to binge eating.

Clinically, when women begin using bioidentical estrogen, they stop gaining weight and often lose 40 percent of the weight they gained since they entered perimenopause. Some women do gain weight on estrogen treatment, but mostly this is a result of water retention. For more information on managing water retention, see the subsection on side effects (page 105).

Studies indicate that bioidentical estradiol in cream form is far more effective in managing weight and insulin sensitivity than the capsule form.

INFLAMMATION PREVENTION

Most women know that inflammation and proinflammatories cause your skin to age prematurely and that eating foods like *wild* salmon, which have high levels of essential fatty acids and other antioxidants (substances that battle the free radicals that cause inflammation), can protect you from this process of deterioration. But did you know that this same destructive inflammation process is responsible for deterioration all over your body? Inflammation promotes many diseases, including arterial sclerosis, cardiovascular disease, arthritis, breast cancer, and even weight gain. Controlling inflammation is paramount to maintaining good health and fighting disease, and bioidentical estrogen is a powerful tool for doing so. Estrogen has significant anti-inflammatory effects, including:

- Estrogen behaves like an antioxidant, controlling free radicals, which cause inflammation.
- Estradiol (E2) decreases two significant promoters of inflammation—interleukin-6 (IL-6) and nuclear factor-kappa B (NF-kB).

Breakthroughs in medicine's understanding of estrogen and its overall disease-fighting power, these studies also explain why one of the earliest symptoms of estrogen deficiency and often the beginning of perimenopause is arthritic-like pain that completely resolves when bioidentical estrogen is supplemented.

BRAIN AND MEMORY SUPPORT

One of the most beneficial aspects of estrogen treatment is its significant protective effect on your cognitive function. Maintaining your estrogen levels protects your memory and brain from age-related deterioration. Failing to do so is devastating to some women's brain function. Have you felt a change in your ability to recall information?

According to Dr. Barbara B. Sherwin, the foremost authority on the subject of estrogen and memory, failing to maintain your estrogen levels may cause a deterioration of your cognitive function—memory loss that cannot be completely regained. If you feel that your memory is not what it used to be, I strongly encourage you to pursue a treatment program, at any age. Because immediate treatment is crucial, I urge you to push past comments like:

"You're too young."
"Let's not do anything drastic."
"Let's wait and see what happens."

Although I support a prudent wait-and-see approach in general medicine, I take seriously Dr. Sherwin's report that in the case of estrogen and memory, failing to take timely action within three to six months may result in irrecoverable loss of memory and brain function that could be avoided by simply restarting an estrogen supplement program. Something *can* and *should* be done to get your memory back to what it was, and perhaps even improve it.

One of the most rewarding aspects of treating women with bioidentical estrogen, is the experience of having women return to the office and tell me the following:

"I can think again!"

"I can remember my lines!"

"I can work without having to write everything down!"

I'm happy to hear patients say this, and always encourage them to share these comments with their other health-care providers to increase other physicians' understanding of why estrogen is important to women beyond their reproductive systems, and at any age. Indeed, since the publication of my last book on the subject of hormones, a tremendous body of scientific data has emerged on the significant health benefits provided by estrogen beyond reproductive function, and particularly to your cognitive function.

If you have complained to your doctor of memory loss and have been told that cognitive function is unrelated to estrogen decline, perimenopause, and menopause, I encourage you to bring the following list to his or her attention. Specifically, estrogen:

- Increases the production of the neurotransmitters acetylcholine, serotonin, and norepinephrine, which help us think and feel.

- Promotes multiple aspects of memory and cognitive function:

  - Increases executive function, also known as cognitive control, which rules logic-based decisions.
  - Increases verbal memory.
  - Increases spatial memory.

- Promotes brain structural health and prevents age-related damage by:

  - Supporting dendrites, the fibers that increase the brain's ability to receive information.
  - Increasing brain-derived neurotrophic factor (BDNF), essential for maintaining brain health.

- Preventing brain gray matter loss, associated with Alzheimer's disease; MRI observation confirmed that postmenopausal women supplementing estrogen enjoyed an increase in gray matter, in contrast to the usual decline associated with aging.
- Protecting against brain white matter loss associated with aging.

• Protects against injury from stroke and epilepsy.

I believe that after presenting this extensive list one would be hard-pressed to deny that estrogen does indeed provide dramatic benefits to memory and cognitive function, nor could one deny the devastating effects of not providing the brain with sufficient levels of estrogen.

DEPRESSION

Estrogen prevents and treats depression; estrogen deficiency causes depression. In fact, when estrogen levels dip down at any stage of life or as a consequence of the natural fluctuation of their monthly cycles, many women often report that they feel depressed, flat, uninspired, and hopeless to varying degrees. See if you can relate to any of the following instances where estrogen deficiency leads to depression or if you know another woman who has:

- Low levels of estrogen in the beginning of a woman's cycle—the days just before and during your period—are associated with depression.
- Women feel less depressed in the second week of their cycles— the week after onset of the period—when estrogen levels rise.
- After delivery, women often experience "baby blues" or even postpartum depression, when estrogen drops dramatically.
- Women in perimenopause—when estrogen declines—experience a greater incidence of depression.
- Depressed women enter menopause at an earlier age.

If these incidents of low mood or depression sound familiar, they should. Estrogen deficiency has been recognized clinically and scientifically as a cause of depression; this cannot be ignored. Unfortunately, it is far more common for women to receive a quick prescription for an antidepressant than a suggestion that she address her estrogen deficiency.

That's really a shame. Treatment with bioidientical estrogen can often alleviate these symptoms. Research has shown that in general, women with depression who do not respond to normal treatments *do* respond to treatment once they supplement estradiol. One study has shown that depressed perimenopausal women who do not respond to conventional therapies with SSRI medications *do* respond when estrogen therapy is incorporated. Also, postpartum depression and postpartum psychosis are successfully treated with estrogen.

Why is estrogen such a strong antidepressant? Specifically, estrogen acts as a monoamine oxidase (MAO) inhibitor, an enzyme that destroys serotonin. Without estrogen, MAO levels are high and serotonin levels fall, leading to depression. It also improves production of serotonin and norepinephrine, which are essential neurotransmitters that help balance mood.

As you can see, estrogen is a natural antidepressant tool that should be used first in treating mood issues, rather than as a last resort.

Rachel's Story

Rachel, forty-nine, a writer, had been on hormone replacement therapy, but was told to stop her treatment by her previous physician after it was thought to be dangerous to women's health. She reported that within a few weeks of stopping her medication, she became *severely* depressed and had even made a suicide attempt. Her whole family was worried about her and she hadn't been able to work since she stopped taking her hormones. She was only able to come to my office because she was accompanied by her husband and writing partner.

(continued)

When we spoke, Rachel reported that she felt depressed, anxious, and that she often hyperventilated and felt shaky. What happened? I explained that her situation was not unique. She was exhibiting the symptoms of estrogen deficiency. In this case, her symptoms were brought on by her abrupt stop to her supplement of estrogen provided by her HRT. In fact, it is common for women to experience a crisis of this nature when they go off their hormone treatment program abruptly or gradually. Estrogen and other hormones do so much more than manage our reproduction, they fuel every aspect of our lives. If you were to abruptly or gradually take gasoline away from an automobile, it would also stop running. What happened to Rachel was the equivalent of putting sugar in a fuel tank—her body was in crisis. I recommended that she gradually reintroduce a bioidentical hormone treatment program that included all three forms of bioidentical estrogen (estrone, estradiol, and estriol, known as E1, E2, and E3), bioidentical progesterone, and 5-Hydroxytryptophan (5-HTP), an amino acid supplement that serves as a natural antidepressant. With this treatment, Rachel gradually improved and within six weeks returned to my office on her own, and reported that she felt even better than she had when treated with nonbioidentical hormones.

ANXIETY AND PANIC ATTACKS

Estrogen prevents and treats anxiety and panic attacks; estrogen deficiency and decline cause anxiety and panic attacks. One of the first signs of declining estrogen is the sudden onset of a panic attack that seems to come from nowhere. These attacks become more frequent in the week before a woman's period and in perimenopause. Bioidentical estrogen treatment has a significant beneficial effect on panic attacks. Studies have found that giving estrogen to women experiencing panic attacks bring these attacks under control. These studies are consistent with my clinical observations. Even for those women in perimenopause, the sooner your panic attacks are treated with bioidentical estrogen, the more effective this remedy can be.

SLEEP

Estrogen promotes sleep and resolves insomnia; estrogen deficiency causes insomnia and poor quality sleep. In fact, one of the first signs of a drop in estrogen levels among perimenopausal women is poor quality sleep. Additionally, women who are many years from perimenopause also experience poor quality sleep in the week before their period, when estrogen levels are low, and better quality sleep in the week following their period, when estrogen levels are relatively high. If you find that you are not sleeping well, or not sleeping at all, I encourage you to consider that you may simply be estrogen deficient, rather than reaching for a chemical sleep medication.

Beyond addressing your insomnia or poor quality sleep directly, treatment with bioidentical estrogen will also help you get to sleep and enjoy better quality sleep in the following ways:

- Insomnia is associated with depression and estrogen helps alleviate depression.
- Insomnia is associated with anxiety and estrogen helps alleviate anxiety.
- Insomnia is associated with migraine headaches, and estrogen helps alleviate headaches.
- Insomnia is associated with night sweats, and estrogen is an effective treatment for night sweats and hot flashes.
- Insomnia is associated with serotonin deficiency, and estrogen increases serotonin levels.

MIGRAINE AND HEADACHE

As discussed in the previous section, estrogen prevents and treats headache and migraine; estrogen deficiency causes headache and migraine. Not all of women's headaches and migraines are related to estrogen deficiency, but many are. For those who suffer from migraines, the headaches occur more frequently on days when estrogen levels decline, like in the week before and during your period, and less frequently in the week after your period, when estrogen is on the rise. Also, migraines and headaches are less common in pregnancy, when estrogen is on the rise and highest. Migraines occur more frequently when estrogen levels drop abruptly—as they do in the placebo week of the birth control pill, when no chemicalized estrogen is provided by the pill, and immediately after the delivery of a child.

If you identify with these patterns of headache and migraine pain, you're not alone. Studies confirm the relationship between migraine headaches and changing levels of estrogen; in fact, these headaches have been termed "menstrual migraines." I encourage you to seek out estrogen treatment as an alternative to simply asking for a prescription for migraine medications.

BONE SUPPORT

Estrogen supports bone strength; estrogen deficiency causes bone loss. Particularly when paired with proper nutritional supplements like magnesium and vitamin D, estrogen treatment offers a safe and effective alternative for medications such as Fosamax and Boniva. For more information on this natural solution to supporting bone strength, see Chapter 16.

SKIN SUPPORT

Estrogen nourishes and hydrates your skin; estrogen deficiency is associated with a pale skin tone and thin, drawn lips. For this reason, treatment with bioidentical estrogen causes women's faces to appear brighter, rounder, and lips fuller and rosier. When applied to the face for three to six months, bioidentical estradiol and estriol in cream form increase elasticity and firmness and decrease wrinkle depth and pore size.

In my practice I offer two compounded face creams—simply called Day Cream and Night Cream—that, in addition to bioidentical estrogen, contain other nutrients that are beneficial to the skin.

Additionally, for women who have a tendency to grow hair on their chin because of intracellular testosterone increase (Chapter 9), applying bioidentical estrogen cream or gel to the affected area may decrease this occurrence.

EYE AND EAR SUPPORT

- **Eyes.** Estrogen offers dramatic benefits for the eyes and for eyesight; estrogen deficiency is associated with deterioration of eyesight. For this reason, treatment with estrogen improves visual function, prevents the increase of eye pressure, associated with glaucoma, and improves the amount and quality of eye lubrication. Failing to correct estrogen deficiency exposes you to an increased risk of general eyesight deterioration, dry-eye syndrome, and glaucoma. Conversely, Premarin, the chemicalized hormone, is associated with higher incidents of dry-eye syndrome.

- **Ears.** Estrogen protects your hearing; estrogen deficiency is associated with age-related hearing loss.

OTHER BENEFITS

- **Muscle development and healing.** Estrogen promotes muscle fiber growth and regeneration; estrogen deficiency is associated with poor muscle development and poor healing rates.

- **Gastrointestinal support.** Estrogen promotes gastrointestinal health; estrogen deficiency increases incidence of duodenal stress ulcers.

- **Energy support.** Estrogen promotes energy; estrogen deficiency increases fatigue, particularly in women with chronic fatigue syndrome (CFS).

ESTROGEN BENEFITS SPECIFIC TO ESTRIOL (E3)

Beyond the benefits of estradiol (E2), estriol (E3) provides a number of unique benefits. Estriol (E3) is the form of estrogen that increases by a thousandfold during pregnancy. More than thirty-five years ago, the protective effects of estriol against breast cancer were established. I never use estradiol (E2) or estrone (E1) without estriol. This combination reflects your own body's preferred estrogen balance, and I believe that in order for it to respond as we'd like, we must respect the notion that a woman's body knows what it requires, and follow suit. In my practice, I use estriol in cream, gel suppository, and sublingual forms. This powerful form of estrogen supports women in the following ways:

- **Restores vaginal integrity.** Estriol is the optimal choice for improvement of vaginal lubrication, resolution of vaginal dryness, and lack of vaginal secretion. When you supplement estriol, you will find that you may not need another lubricant. A large number of women—many not in menopause and perimenopause—experience vaginal dryness, in some cases related to their use of oral contraceptives or a relatively low level of estrogen. Estriol is able to completely restore the unique ecosystem of the vagina, restoring the elasticity and rebuilding the tissue of the vaginal walls, increasing production of friendly bacteria, and by doing so decreasing urinary tract infection (UTI), vaginal infection, and future stress incontinence or prolapse of the vaginal walls.

  Estriol does not promote uterine tissue growth and may even decrease the proliferation of uterine lining, which may decrease the incidence of uterine cancer.

- **Alleviates night sweats and hot flashes.** Estriol is able to quickly, effectively, and safely resolve both night sweats and hot flashes in the absolute majority of women. Simply remedying this annoyance allows many women to finally get a good night's sleep.

- **Decreases inflammation.** Estriol has a significant anti-inflammatory effect. It decreases nuclear factor-kappa beta (NFkB), a primary inflammation marker, tumor necrosis factor-alpha (TNF-a), and inflammation that specifically affects osteoporosis.

- **Improvement in multiple sclerosis (MS).** The most significant anti-inflammatory effect of estriol is in multiple sclerosis (MS), a chronic neuron-degenerative disease that is often diagnosed in young women. Again, in pregnancy, estriol levels increase a thousandfold. While they are pregnant, most MS patients improve significantly without other treatment. In my practice, I have successfully used bioidentical estriol to treat women with MS for more than ten years. Only one medical center publishes reports about the treatment of MS with bioidentical estriol. In its reports, the UCLA Medical Center reported tremendously successful results using MRI imaging to demonstrate positive changes in the brains of the women studied. Why wouldn't everyone use this simple and inexpensive treatment for this destructive disease that affects so many young women?

- **Breast cancer protection.** The most dramatic and beneficial use of estriol is likely in the field of the prevention and possible treatment of breast cancer. Two estrogen receptors are found in the breast, alpha and beta. These receptors are the parts of the cell that enable estrogen to express its function. The alpha receptors affect the growth of breast tissue—both normal and abnormal, while beta receptors suppress the growth of both types of breast tissue. Estradiol affects the function of both alpha and beta receptors, meaning, it concurrently affects the growth of breast tissue, including unwanted abnormal tissue, and the decrease of this tissue. By contrast, estriol affects only the beta receptors, which means it suppresses the growth of only the (normal and) abnormal breast tissue. In addition, estriol specifically prevents breast cancer cells from producing new blood vessels by blocking vascular endothelial growth factor (VEGF), a protein that promotes the spread of the cancer.

I encourage any reader who is told by her physician that she does not need to supplement estriol because it is so weak relative to the other two forms of estrogen, and therefore is not important, to submit this information and fully avail herself of the power of this "little" hormone.

HOW TO SUPPLEMENT ESTROGEN

 Lili's Story

Lili, thirty-five, a stay-at-home mom, visited me and reported that she was already on bioidentical hormone replacement therapy for the treatment of premenstrual syndrome. She reported only minimal benefits, in spite of the fact that her saliva test indicated that her hormone levels had increased significantly. Lili wanted to know why she didn't feel better. I explained that saliva tests should never be a monitoring tool for bioidentical use. The most minimal hormone supplementation significantly raises the level of hormone measured in saliva, and prevents the proper treatment based on how a woman actually feels. I checked Lili's blood levels for estrogen and progesterone, which were very low, despite the adequate dose of hormones in the cream treatment she used. To correct this, I recommended that Lili switch to a gel treatment, which in my experience has a significantly better absorption rate. This switch raised Lili's hormone levels in a meaningful way, allowing her to feel the benefits of her bioidentical HRT treatment.

Forms of Estrogen

Bioidentical estrogen supplements come in five delivery systems: transdermal (cream or gel applied to skin), sublingual (drops or pill placed under the tongue), internal (vaginal suppositories), oral (pill or capsule swallowed), and injectable. Each of these enters your body in a different way, to various degrees of efficacy. Some delivery forms are better for the treatment of certain conditions than others. Following is a discussion of the forms of estrogen and their suitability to treating your symptoms.

Additionally, this section also addresses what type of the three forms of estrogen are needed—estrone (E1), estradiol (E2), or estriol (E3)—how supplementing one form affects the other two, and which delivery systems help you achieve the balance of all three estrogens that allows you to safely achieve your supplement goals.

Transdermal Cream or Gel

At least 90 percent of my patients who use bioidentical estrogen use the cream or gel form, by applying it to the skin on their inner arms and thighs and the palms of their hands. I favor the delivery of estrogen by this mechanism because it absorbs well, brings estrogen levels up evenly, so that they peak within three hours, and maintains levels for ten to twenty-four hours. As patients get to know their needs for estrogen, this form also allows them to easily modify their dosage by using more or less cream or gel, more often or less often throughout the day. Other transdermal options, like the patch, do not allow for these modifications. The great majority of my patients must use their cream or gel twice a day. Some use it more than twice a day.

Another reason I favor cream or gel forms is that they do not significantly affect women's sex-binding globulin levels. When sex-binding globulin increases, it decreases the effective levels of other hormones available to you. Additionally, creams and gels do not increase the incidence of blood clots in your cardiovascular system, and are least compromising to breast support efforts. The cream or gel form is called "triest," and includes all three forms of estrogen—E1, E2, and E3.

Setting your dose. The dose of the *triest* estrogen cream or gel I use in my practice contains:

2.5 mg of estriol
0.75 mg of estradiol
0.25 mg of estrone, per gram of cream or gel

Results are highly individual and depend on symptom resolution and blood testing. In my practice, patients use as little as one-eighth of a gram, once a day, to as much as 1 or 2 grams several times a day. Every woman requires a different dose to treat different symptoms, because every woman's body absorbs the ingredients in the cream or gel to a different degree.

Special uses for estriol cream or gel. On page 96, I discuss the unique benefits of supplementing estriol (E3), the "little" estrogen that can do so much. To treat the symptoms described in this section, I recommend a cream or gel that only contains estriol and is applied vaginally, To increase vaginal lubrication, I suggest that patients apply the cream or gel, internally, but only as far as the first two inches inside the vagina. This improves vaginal lubrication but does not allow the estriol to absorb into the bloodstream and disturb your estrogen balance.

I recommend patients apply estriol beyond the first two inches of the vagina to treat infertility, stress incontinence, and other conditions. The estriol cream or gel I use contains 1 to 2 mg of estriol for every 1 gram of cream or gel. In my practice, patients use ranges from a half to 2 mg daily. Remember, creams and gels are not all the same. If you find that the cream or gel you use fails to remedy your condition despite your high dose, it may be that the product you are using is not penetrating your vaginal wall to the extent necessary to provide you with benefits.

Fine tuning. Although creams and gels are effective, there are nonetheless two problems typical to the use of this delivery form:

- **Skin irritation and occasional rash at the site of application** and rarely in other areas. I believe that this is a reaction to the component used in the cream that aids in hormone absorption. Over the years I have worked together with the various compounding pharmacists who serve my patient population to develop creams and gels that are hypoallergenic. There is still a minority of women for whom this problem persists regardless of how mild the formula. For these women I recommend sublingual drops.

- **Poor absorption rates in varying formulas.** Because the formulas of compounding pharmacies differ from pharmacy to pharmacy, I often see patients who use a cream or gel that yields a low hormone absorption rate. Because I am a believer in this treatment modality, I have devoted a great deal of time and thought to the development of the compounded form of the cream and gel that I recommend to my patients. These creams and gels offer the best absorption rate I have seen. Of course, there remains a group of women for whom creams and gels do not work; for these women, I recommend sublingual drops.

USING CREAM OR GEL TO PREVENT AND REMEDY HEADACHE AND MIGRAINE

A drop in estrogen levels before or during your period, and sometimes in the middle of your cycle, can trigger headache and migraine. In my practice, I have had great success in using bioidentical estrogen cream or gel to treat women with these problems. However, this treatment can only be effective if bioidentical estrogen is supplemented *before* your actual drop in estrogen levels. If you supplement estrogen after the drop begins, you will only enjoy a mild benefit. A physician with experience in treatment with bioidentical estrogen can help you identify the optimum days for you to begin increasing your natural level of estrogen.

(continued)

In my clinical experience, applying estrogen gel or cream directly on the area that is causing the headache pain can sometimes provide additional relief.

The advantage to using bioidentical estrogen over prescription medications in the triptan group to treat headache and migraine is that bioidentical estrogen is able to prevent the onset of these headaches, whereas triptan medications don't, and are only helpful in alleviating pain in the first few hours of the migraine.

SUBLINGUAL DROPS

Some patients develop an allergic reaction to estrogen cream or gel, or decide that they would rather not wait for these products to dry before they get dressed. Many of these women prefer to use sublingual drops, even though they are not ideal hormone delivery systems. Taking your estrogen sublingually causes your estradiol levels to peak quickly and then drop just as fast, leaving your bloodstream entirely in six to eight hours. In addition, this form of supplementation increases sex-binding globulin. Because of its short duration of effectiveness, it must be used more than twice a day, in many cases as often as four times a day. The sublingual form of estradiol also increases estrone levels. As explained, ideally, estradiol and estrone are found in equal amounts in the blood. When estradiol is supplemented sublingually, blood tests indicate that the level of estrone rises far higher than estradiol. For this reason, when taking estradiol sublingually, you need not supplement estrone, but you should absolutely supplement estriol. This combination of estradiol and estriol is called "biest" (meaning, two estrogens).

Estradiol sublinguals versus biest sublingual. I am aware of a number of physicians who recommend the sublingual use of estradiol (E2) alone as a primary form of estrogen treatment. I am concerned about the use of estradiol without estriol (E3), the form of estrogen that balances E2 and protects women from the consequences of unbalanced estrogen. Of all the estrogen delivery systems, the use of sublingual estradiol, more than all others, requires the accompaniment of estriol.

> In my practice, I limit my recommendation of sublingual biest (estradiol and estriol) for the treatment of specific conditions intermittently and on a short-term basis, or in situations where I believe it is necessary to increase a patient's sex-binding globulin in order to manage unwanted symptoms in patients with high levels of testosterone. These unwanted side effects include acne, head hair loss, and facial hair growth. I may also recommend sublingual biest in cases where a patient has sensitive skin and develops a rash by using a cream or gel.

Setting your dose. In my practice, patients use one to six drops, two to four times daily. Each drop contains 0.5 mg of estriol and 0.1 mg of estradiol.

I recommend estriol drops for the treatment of conditions described on pages 96 to 98 in women who are unable to absorb estriol in cream or gel form. Each drop contains 1 mg of estriol. My patients use one to eight drops, two or three times daily.

Suppositories

I recommend vaginal estriol suppositories for patients who seek to increase their vaginal lubrication. Each suppository contains 2 mg of estriol; patients insert one suppository into the first two inches of the vagina before going to sleep.

Capsules or Pills

In my practice, I rarely recommend the use of capsules and pills for the following reasons. Capsules and pills:

- Must be processed by the liver, which is taxing on the organ and also increases sex-binding globulin, which can limit the availability of other hormones.
- Increase inflammation by increasing C-reactive protein (CRP), a general indicator of inflammation.
- May increase blood clots.
- May not be as favorable to breast tissue.
- Overall, have unfavorable absorption rates.

Setting your dose. In my practice, I use these forms as the delivery systems of last resort. I do so with the following dosing modifications:

As explained, under ideal circumstances, estradiol and estrone are found at equal amounts in blood. When estradiol is taken in pill or capsule form by mouth, blood tests indicate that the level of estrone rises far higher than estradiol. For this reason, when taking estradiol in pill and capsule form, you need not supplement estrone, but you should absolutely supplement estriol. As mentioned above, in my office I use a biest capsule that combines 0.1 mg estradiol and 0.5 mg of estriol. Patients use one to five capsules, twice daily.

INJECTIBLE

Bioidentical estradiol is also available in pellets that are injected just under the skin (subdermal). I do not use this delivery method in my practice because it requires an in-office surgical procedure and causes estradiol levels to rise and sustain their level for one to three months. Once absorbed, this method does not allow you to decrease the level of estradiol delivered. As discussed, women must be able to modify their intake of estrogen, in some cases on a daily basis.

THE ESTRADIOL PATCH

Estradiol is also available as a transdermal patch from traditional pharmacies. However, I prefer to use a compounding pharmacy cream or gel for transdermal application for the following reasons:

- **No patch contains estriol.** I don't recommend estradiol without estriol. You'll find additional information on the benefits of this combination in the sections that follow.

- **The patch controls you; you do not control the patch.** Its single-dose option does not give you the opportunity to adjust your dose in the event that your optimal dose of estradiol is more or less than the uniform dose chosen for you. Moreover, in the start of this estrogen section, I presented data to support why the low-dose patch does not provide you with the benefits you may be using the patch for. Finally, although the patch is designed to deliver a specific and reliable dose, studies have shown that the patch delivers unpredictable amounts.

- **Not powerful enough for full benefit.** For many women, even the highest-dose patch does not deliver enough estrogen to resolve all their symptoms.

In addition, patients complain that the patch can sometimes fall off midday. Finally, unlike a cream or gel that is invisible once absorbed, the patch and its outline are visible, preventing some patients from wearing what they like.

Possible Side Effects

- **Water retention** is the most common side effect associated with supplementing bioidentical estrogen. It takes two to five days to appear, and just as long to resolve. It may present itself as swollen legs, weight gain, breast or nipple pain, or swollen hands, fingers, and feet and ankles. Simply decreasing the amount of estrogen used generally resolves this condition. You may reduce your dose and you no longer experience breast pain, but overall, you feel less well because you are not receiving as much estrogen. If so, in my practice, I recommend using herbal and nutrition supplements that act as natural diuretics to allow patients to increase their estrogen levels without experiencing water retention. If your water retention is expressed as breast pain alone, consider switching to a bra that does not include an underwire, or not wearing a bra at all. For more information on how wearing a bra can affect the way your breasts feel and your overall breast health, see Chapter 17.

One explanation for water retention experienced by women who supplement estrogen is that some women have a biological tendency to produce a large amount of estrone sulfate (ES), a natural reservoir of estrogen. In the case of these women, when ES increases, the benefits they enjoy from supplementing estrogen decrease. A physician with experience in the treatment with bioidentical hormones can advise you on individual remedies for this condition.

- **Abnormal bleeding** may occur for a number of reasons. You may be taking too much, or too little, estrogen; you may be taking too much, or too little, progesterone. A physician who has experience with bioidentical hormones will help you find the perfect balance needed to resolve this abnormal bleeding. Or there may be a potential abnormality in the uterus itself. Any incidence of pelvic bleeding should be evaluated by your gynecologist utilizing pelvic ultrasound.

- **Hot flashes** may occur in the earliest stages of treatment. This simply means that more estrogen receptors are opening. As you gradually increase your dose of bioidentical estrogen, these hot flashes will resolve.

Overuse is another reason for experiencing hot flashes while using bioidentical estrogen. When you have exceeded your ideal dose of bioidentical estrogen, a type of "estrogen flooding" occurs, where too much estrogen is competing for estrogen receptors. Simply reducing your dose will resolve this effect.

- **Opposite-from-expected response** may also occur when supplementing bioidentical estrogen in unusual cases, just as with any other bioidentical hormone. Examples of this type of effect include experiencing poor sleep rather than better sleep, acne breakouts rather than helping your skin clear up, aggressive feelings rather than calm and patience, and other reactions that are the direct opposite of the reason you sought out bioidentical estrogen in the first place. A physician with experience in treatment with bioidentical hormones can advise you on individual remedies for each of these conditions.

BRAIN AND MEMORY SUPPORT

Common hormone-based memory remedies to avoid

Confusion and, in some cases, erroneous news about the damage that estrogen can do to your body, combined with scientific data about how essential estrogen is to women's cognitive function, has led to the development of weak, middle-ground solutions that will not improve the conditions of women who go to the trouble of using them. Specifically:

- **Low-dose transdermal estradiol patch.** This low-dose patch provides too little estradiol to benefit cognitive function.

- **Intermittent dosing.** Another useless middle-ground solution is the recommendation that women use their estrogen intermittently, every other day or twice a week, for example. Studies indicated that

(continued)

supplementing estrogen intermittently impairs, rather than helps, cognition.

- **Very low-dose birth control pills.** Although there has been a general trend of developing low-dose birth control pills for many years, the recent scares about estrogen and HRT have caused manufacturers to further reduce the dose of chemicalized estrogen in oral contraceptives. When women take birth control pills, the pill shuts down all natural ovarian estrogen and progesterone production. When women use super-low-dose oral contraceptives, they are effectively put into an estrogen-deficient state. Studies indicate that birth control pill users have a decline in cognition. In my practice, I regularly observe that women—even young women—who use this new generation of very-low-dose birth control pills exhibit frequent memory loss.

I urge you to think twice before deciding to forgo bioidentical estrogen or use one of the ineffective low-dose methods described above.

5 • Progesterone: Estrogen's Best Friend

QUICK QUIZ

Answer the following questions to see if you might be experiencing a progesterone deficiency:

Do you have irregular periods?

Have you stopped getting a period altogether?

Do you spot before your period?

Are your menstrual cramps worse than in years past?

Have your periods gotten heavier?

Do you experience premenstrual breast pain? Breast size increase?

Do you experience premenstrual water retention?

Have you been told that you may have endometriosis?

Have you been diagnosed with having fibroids?

Are you more nervous premenstrually?

(continued)

Do you experience poor quality sleep before and during your period?

Do you find that you are less calm than you used to be, in general?

Have birth control pills been recommended to you as a way to "regulate" your cycle?

If you relate to any of these conditions during part or all of the month, you are experiencing the symptoms of progesterone deficiency or partial progesterone deficiency.

Lisa's Story

Lisa, thirty-eight, reported that for the last three years she has been retaining more and more water premenstrually, she feels more anxious, her breasts have grown a full cup size, and her periods have been progressively getting heavier. Her previous physician recommended that she take birth control pills to remedy her complaints. Lisa requested that he test her blood to measure hormone levels prior to her beginning the medication, and, although he was not enthusiastic about doing so, he finally agreed.

Lisa's birth control pill treatment did decrease her menstrual flow, but also increased her weight and water retention, and caused her breasts to feel heavier and more painful all month long; she also felt more anxious and even less sexual. By the time I saw Lisa in my office, she was really at her wit's end. A review of the original blood tests performed by her previous physician before she began her birth control pill treatment revealed far from optimal progesterone levels. And although her previous doctor had faithfully followed mainstream medicine's indicated course of treatment, to me it made no sense from a hormonal perspective. Rather than giving Lisa bioidentical progesterone to optimize her relative lower levels, the birth control pill recommendation *eliminated all* of Lisa's natural progesterone production in favor of supplementing it with a chemical. How can this be better for her? I recommended that Lisa stop taking the birth control pills and begin taking bioidentical progesterone.

Within three months, Lisa's original complaints and new pill-related side effects had completely resolved.

Michelle's Story: Other Reasons for Abnormal Bleeding

Michelle, thirty-eight, began having irregular periods and once missed a whole cycle. She was previously prescribed birth control pills to remedy this and regulate her cycle. She reported that no other questions were asked about why her periods were irregular—she was simply handed a prescription. In the first three months after beginning taking this medication, she gained fifteen pounds and reports that she lost a great majority of her sex drive. In addition, she would get severe migraine headaches on the day she began her placebo pill (day twenty-one of her cycle). When she reported this to her previous health-care provider, she was told to skip the placebo pills altogether and begin a new birth control pack on day twenty-one, when she would have begun her placebo series. Once she implemented this recommendation her headaches did stop, but she gained another five pounds in the subsequent first month and reports that she became completely inorgasmic. Her blood workup indicated an abnormal result in her thyroid function test, which was further aggravated by the birth control pills prescribed. I recommended that she stop taking the birth control pills and, instead, supplement her thyroid function with bioidentical thyroid. Within three months of making these changes, Michelle's periods were regulated, she shed the weight she had put on as a consequence of the birth control pill treatment, and resumed her sexual desire and function.

PROGESTERONE BASICS

Although many women don't realize it, progesterone is the second most important hormone that makes you the woman you are. Progesterone helps you realize your goal of becoming pregnant, if you choose to. It also balances the role of estrogen to ensure that you are able to function with energy and a positive mood by making you soft and calm, yet allows you to feel in control of yourself, your surroundings, and your challenges. Progesterone additionally balances the work of estrogen to keep you disease free.

Progesterone Benefits

Progesterone directly provides the following lifestyle improvements and disease-prevention properties:

- **Breast cancer protection.** One of the most important roles of progesterone is that it protects you from breast cancer; progesterone deficiency increases your risk of breast cancer. More specifically, optimized levels of progesterone protect you from breast cancer by:

  - Converting estradiol (E2) to estrone (E1), the far weaker form of estrogen, which helps maintain a proper estrogen balance.
  - Balancing the effect of estrogen by decreasing estrogen receptors, increasing their rate of breakdown, and decreasing their rate of buildup, all important to preventing the development of cancer.
  - Increasing P53, a natural substance that protects the body from breast cancer and blocks BCL–2, a substance that increases cancer.
  - Blocking urokinase plasminogen activator, a natural substance that increases the proliferation of cancer.
  - Additionally blocking the cascade of events that trigger and fuel breast cancer, including the blocking of nuclear factor-kappa beta (NFkB) and COX-2.

- Protecting breast tissue from HER-2/neu oncogene, an aggressive breast cancer marker, present in 30 percent of all women with breast cancer.

Every one of the actions above make a dramatic difference in the direction of breast cancer development, and each is controlled or decreased by bioidentical progesterone. For this reason, it is imperative that women optimize their progesterone levels and include bioidentical progesterone in any other hormone treatment program, in order to balance the effect of these hormones and generally protect their breast tissue from the development of cancer.

STUDIES SUPPORT PROGESTERONE'S POWER TO FIGHT BREAST CANCER

In clinical studies, progesterone has been shown to protect from breast cancer.

- In a recent study, a postmenopausal group taking estradiol with bioidentical progesterone was compared with a second group taking estradiol and Provera. All cancer biomarkers that were tested had increased in the group taking Provera, while none had increased in the group taking progesterone.

- In studies on women operated on to remove breast cancer, those women who were operated on during the days in their cycles when their bodies produce progesterone (days fifteen to twenty-eight) enjoyed an overall increased survival rate, as compared with women who had surgery at other times in their cycle.

- A study of 1,150 French women who used bioidentical progesterone cream on their breasts to decrease breast pain found that those who

(continued)

used bioidentical progesterone enjoyed an overall decrease in incidence of breast cancer.

- In an unprecedented study at Johns Hopkins Medical Center conducted on 1,083 women over thirty years, two distinct groups—one
  group with low progesterone and one group with normal progesterone—found that the low progesterone group had a 5.4-fold
  higher incidence of perimenopausal breast cancer, a tenfold higher
  mortality rate from cancer in general, and a threefold higher mortality rate from all causes. Aren't these numbers shocking? A low level of
  naturally occurring progesterone in these women's bodies translated
  into threefold more deaths, tenfold more deaths from cancer, and
  more than fivefold incidence of breast cancer.

- Also, a recent French study on 54,000 women compared nonusers,
  bioidentical progesterone users, and chemical Progestatin users. As
  compared to nonusers, the group that used chemical Progestin experienced an increase in incidence of breast cancer. The group that used
  bioidentical progesterone enjoyed a 10 percent decrease in breast cancer as compared to the nonuser group. The latest French study on this
  subject compared nonusers to a group that used bioidentical estrogen
  and progesterone and followed up these groups for an average of eight
  years. The study observed that those women who used no hormones
  suffered a sixfold higher incidence of breast cancer, as compared to the
  group that used bioidentical estrogen and progesterone.

These and other clinical studies establish that your body produces progesterone to protect your breasts. I strongly urge women to question
those who say that women do not need progesterone, and further question those who suggest the supplement of estrogen without also supplementing bioidentical progesterone. For a more detailed discussion of
how progesterone helps prevent breast cancer, see Chapter 17.

> **Special note for women on hormone-based birth control:** Are you on the pill? Whether you realize it or not, you are also on hormone replacement therapy. I caution the millions of women who currently use chemical-based contraception—whether in the form of pills, patches, or vaginal rings—that these birth control means have the same problems associated with chemicalized "hormone" medications. The pill, the patch, and rings all shut off your natural production of progesterone in favor of chemicals in these products.

Cardiac health. Earlier we discussed how bioidentical estrogen supports your cardiovascular health; progesterone protects you from cardiac-related health problems by inhibiting vascular cell adhesion molecule 1 (VCAM–1), an inflammation factor involved in the process of arterial sclerosis.

- **Brain support.** Like estrogen, progesterone promotes the function and maintenance of the brain. In addition, progesterone has also been shown to be protective of the peripheral nerve system that includes the spine by increasing the production of myelin, the fatty substance that creates a cushion around our peripheral nerve system. This benefit explains why the condition of women with multiple sclerosis improves during pregnancy, when progesterone levels shoot up a hundred-fold. Progesterone significantly aids in recovery from brain trauma by decreasing edema, or swelling in the brain.

- **Anxiety, depression, and other mood conditions.** If you feel anxious, panicked, or experience hyperventilation or stress, progesterone helps alleviate these conditions by increasing your production of GABA, the neurotransmitter that allows you to feel calm and relaxed. Women who are given the opportunity to use progesterone to treat their anxiety report the following:

"It's a lifesaver."
"It works like magic."
"I've never felt so calm."

One recent study followed 176 women who were given Provera for five years and switched to bioidentical progesterone for six months. After switching, they reported a significant improvement in mood, and decrease in anxiety and depression.

And unlike other medications that alleviate anxiety and depression, bioidentical progesterone is never addictive.

For specific recommendations on treating anxiety, depression, and other mood conditions with progesterone, see Part Three, on the mind and mood pillar.

Additionally, bioidentical progesterone dramatically improves the condition of women suffering from postpartum depression and "baby blues." For more information on this subject, please see my extensive recommendations in *How to Make a New Mother Happy* (Chronicle Books).

- **Sleep.** Progesterone helps you fall asleep, stay asleep, and improve the quality of sleep. Progesterone increases your production of the "feel-good" neurotransmitter GABA. In my clinical experience this treatment alone is often enough to resolve complaints of poor sleep and insomnia.

- **Other benefits.** As if all of the benefits listed in this chapter weren't enough, optimizing your progesterone levels provides you with the following direct benefits:

  - Improves immunity.
  - Builds bones.

- Improves hearing.
- Protects from seizures.
- Decreases allergies.
- Decreases irritable bowel syndrome (IBS).
- Decreases interstitial cystitis.
- Prevents and resolves water retention.

How to Supplement Progesterone

Available forms and efficacy. Bioidentical progesterone comes in capsules, sublingual drops, and cream. Sublingual drops produce a quick rise in progesterone blood levels within a half hour, but these levels drop to pretreatment levels within six to ten hours. For this reason, sublingual drops are ideal for conditions when you require a quick effect—falling asleep, alleviating anxiety and irritation, and other conditions that require short-term results. Note that this means that you will have to use these drops three to four times daily to maintain your desired effect.

CAPSULES

In capsule form, bioidentical progesterone peaks in blood levels within two to four hours and lasts for ten to fourteen hours. I recommend splitting your intended dose so that you take a higher dose at night and a lower dose during the day in order to insure that you don't become sleepy.

Concerns about Prometrium gelcaps. Bioidentical progesterone is available in a variety of doses from compounding pharmacies, but is also available through conventional pharmacies under the brand name Prometrium. My concern about Prometrium is that it contains peanut oil and is only available in relatively high doses. For this reason, most women choose to take Prometrium during the night, as the high dose causes them to feel sleepy if taken during the day. The problem with restricting your dosage to evening is that within twelve hours the majority of Prometrium leaves your system, limiting your body to the benefits of progesterone for only twelve out of the twenty-four hours of each day. For this reason I prefer the wide spectrum of individualized doses available from compounding pharmacies. See the Resources section at the back of the book for more information on compounding pharmacies.

CREAM

Bioidentical progesterone cream is widely used and has a much milder effect on mind, mood, and sleep. When using creams the increase in progesterone blood levels is relatively low. Low doses of bioidentical progesterone cream are available over the counter, without a prescription, but these lowest doses are often not sufficient to balance estrogen treatment, as described in the previous section. Whether you source your bioidentical progesterone from a compounding pharmacy, conventional pharmacy, or over the counter, your use should be constantly monitored by your gynecologist.

Setting your dose: In my practice, the dosage of progesterone I recommend to my patients varies widely, based on the condition to be treated and the patient's starting progesterone level. Dosage may be as low as 10 mg daily to as high as 400 mg daily. A physician with experience in recommending bioidentical hormones can help you determine the individual dose that will best suit your goals.

Using progesterone as a sleep aid. To help you fall asleep and improve sleep quality, begin with a starter dose of 10 mg daily and increase your dose daily until you reach a dose that resolves your sleep challenges. Reduce this dose if you experience the side effects described in the section that follows. If you find that you fall asleep but then wake up in the middle of the night, you may use half of the dose that helped you get to sleep in the first place. When you awake in the morning, be mindful of how you feel, as a common side effect of using too much progesterone is dizziness.

For specific recommendations on treating sleep challenges with progesterone, see Chapter 14.

DOES NATURE WANT WOMEN TO MAINTAIN THEIR PERIODS FOREVER?

We live in a strange new era. Although nature has determined that the menstrual cycle should end at the conclusion of menopause, a vocal group has challenged nature, claiming that women ought to use bioidentical progesterone in a way that allows them to continue having periods indefinitely. Proponents of this philosophy report:

"It makes me feel young."

"It's natural."

"It helps me detox."

At its most basic, a menstrual period is the body's reaction to a failure to conceive that also prepares your body for another chance to do so in the subsequent month. But at no time in human history prior to the last hundred years have women had a lifetime's worth of regular periods. The "natural" life of a woman meant that she spent the years between puberty and menopause mostly pregnant or lactating, with very few weeks of menstrual flow. Anthropologists estimate that women living in this way had less than fifty periods in their *entire lives*.

I have seen the medical consequences of women living with limited lifetime periods, firsthand. Between 1972 and 1976, I worked as a gynecologist in a rural part of Israel. Most of the women who lived in this area had never practiced any form of birth control and used constant procreation and breastfeeding as a continuous, natural lifestyle. In many cases this meant they had twelve to twenty children to raise. Despite their exhaustion, they were healthier; did not experience PMS, endometriosis, painful periods, or breast pain; and had only a relatively low incidence of breast cancer, uterine cancer, and ovarian cancer.

I am not suggesting that women ought to have more children than they feel comfortable bearing, nor am I suggesting that women who

(continued)

choose not to have children are jeopardizing their health. What I am proposing is that once you understand all of the benefits associated with optimizing your progesterone levels (as happens without supplementation in pregnancy), I believe that you will choose to maintain your use of progesterone throughout the month starting with perimenopause and for the optimal number of days throughout the month prior to perimenopause.

Possible Side Effects

- **Minor side effects.** The most common side effect associated with supplementing bioidentical progesterone is an overproduction of the neurotransmitter GABA, which may cause you to feel sleepy, dizzy, and have a feeling similar to being intoxicated. This side effect can be felt as soon as a half hour and can last as long as eight hours after your dose is taken. To resolve this, simply reduce your dose or switch your supplement method to a cream.

- **Opposite-from-expected effects.** As with all bioidentical hormones, in some cases bioidentical progesterone treatment yields a response that is the exact opposite of what you expect. In general, this occurs more frequently the older you are. Paradoxical effects include:

  - **Sign of estrogen deficiency,** including poor mood, hot flashes, headaches, feelings of panic, and memory loss. This occurs when your progesterone supplement blocks or decreases your supply of estrogen. A physician who has experience with bioidentical hormones will recognize this effect and recommend steps for resolution.
  - **Increased agitation,** as the result of a higher-than-preferred cortisol level. This happens when progesterone blocks an enzyme called 11-beta-hydroxysteroid, which is meant to convert cortisol to cortisone, the inactive form of cortisol. When the work of

11-beta-hydroxysteroid is blocked, your level of cortisol rises and you experience agitation rather than the usual calming effect associated with progesterone.

- **Water retention,** which can occur when the rise of cortisol over-comes the diuretic effect of progesterone. Progesterone is a strong antagonist of the adrenal hormone aldosterone, which causes water retention. Because progesterone battles against aldosterone, progesterone also works as a natural diuretic. However, some-times when the significant increase of cortisol within the cell described above occurs, women nonetheless experience water re-tention, breast pain, and water weight gain. A physician experi-enced with bioidentical hormones will recognize this effect and recommend steps for resolution.

- **Toxic response,** something very few women will feel when using even the smallest dose of progesterone. Their blood pressure falls, they hyperventilate, they feel panicked, and their pulse rises. These women may have chronic viral syndrome, Lyme disease, toxic effect of black mold and heavy metals, severe environmental aller-gies, or an increase of yeast growth. Until these conditions are treated and resolved, these women will remain among the very few who are not able to enjoy the benefits of bioidentical progesterone.

Using Progesterone and the Four Pillars for Specific Conditions

Progesterone is essential for the treatment of symptoms of PMS, irreg-ular bleeding, the painful periods associated with endometriosis and cycle-related fertility issues. In the following sections I address how you can use progesterone supplements and the four pillars to naturally resolve all of these health challenges.

- **Premenstrual syndrome (PMS).** Ironically, PMS was never consid-ered to be a bona fide medical condition until the medication Prozac was approved for the "treatment" of PMS. As a gynecologist with many years of focus on women's wellness, I can assure you that no woman with PMS suffers from Prozac deficiency, but these women do have hormonal and nutritional deficiencies. In my clinical experience, any emotional or physical changes that occur within the window of time starting as early as two weeks before your period, through the duration of your period, whether short or long, mild or severe, should be characterized as PMS.

- **PMS basics.** PMS symptoms have three components:

  - **Subjective signs of estrogen deficiency.** You feel flat, uninspired, depressed, and experience panic, mood swings, insomnia, memory loss, and migraine. The closer you get to the start of your period, the worse these symptoms become.
  - **Subjective signs of progesterone deficiency.** You experience water retention, breast and nipple pain, anxiousness, and agitation. The closer you get to the start of your period, the worse these symptoms become.
  - **Subjective signs of increased testosterone.** Aggressive behavior, impatience, short-temperedness, development of acne, and oily skin. The closer you get to the start of your period, the worse these symptoms become.

In the past, most women diagnosed with PMS were younger and had progesterone deficiency. For these women, supplementing bioidentical progesterone provided significant benefits and relief. At this time, a non-medical term called "estrogen dominance" became popular, erroneously postulating that high estrogen levels caused PMS and effectively scaring women away from bioidentical estrogen. Although long ago discredited, this term continues to be used by some out-of-date health-care providers. The truth is, these women did not have too much estrogen, they simply didn't have enough progesterone. In the last ten years I have seen a growing number of women who have adequate levels of progesterone but have relatively lower-than-expected levels of estrogen.

Using Progesterone and the Four Pillars to Treat PMS

HORMONE BALANCE PRINCIPLES TO TREAT PMS

- **Progesterone.** I have used bioidentical progesterone to treat PMS with great success for more than twenty-five years, but standard medical protocols have yet to acknowledge this tool as a method of treatment.

  The younger you are, the more likely it is that simply supplementing bioidentical progesterone will resolve your PMS symptoms. Studies have shown that women with PMS have low levels of progesterone and its metabolite allopregnenolone.

  In the treatment of PMS, the use of bioidentical progesterone in sublingual drops and pill form is significantly more effective than the cream form. The ideal dose is extremely individualized, and there is no barrier to how high a dose you can take so long as you continue to enjoy benefits. Your dose should be reduced when a higher one fails to yield additional benefits, if the higher dose yields *fewer* benefits, or if you experience the side effects described in the sections that follow.

- **Estrogen.** As mentioned earlier, over the last ten years I have observed that less than optimal estrogen levels in women with PMS have become a growing contributor to this condition. During this time frame, I also noticed that my course of treatment with bioidentical progesterone alone was less effective in treating both PMS and postpartum depression. I was puzzled. Then in 1995 I saw a scientific article showing the benefit of supplementing bioidentical estrogen for the treatment of PMS. Since then I have successfully incorporated bioidentical estrogen into my treatment of PMS and postpartum depression—with and without progesterone—with great outcomes. Recently, two additional articles have emphasized the important role of decreased levels of estrogen in the causation of PMS.

In my practice, I recommend using bioidentical estrogen in cream form, with application beginning at the onset of symptoms and the amount you apply increasing in the days leading up to your period, as your symptoms increase. I generally continue treatment through the third or fourth day of the menstrual period and then suggest that cream application taper off over a few days.

• **Testosterone.** Three common symptoms of PMS are oily skin, acne, and aggressive behavior, all signs of more pronounced testosterone expression. This rise in testosterone occurs within the cells and is therefore imperceptible in blood testing. For this reason we say that there is a rise in testosterone expression, rather than levels. Why does this happen? Your cycle's decrease in estrogen also decreases sex-binding globulin, a protein generally charged with binding testosterone. With both of these powerful monitors less present, testosterone expresses itself more dominantly, causing oily skin, breakouts, and aggressive behavior.

Treatment for the symptoms associated with an increased expression of testosterone should not include birth control pills or other medications that "block" the effects of testosterone. Instead, I recommend simply following your body's own example and increasing estrogen levels (and therefore sex-binding globulin levels) by treatment with bioidentical estrogen. Particularly in the case of young women, the dose of estrogen used should start at the very minimum and increase extremely slowly, as even a dose that is a bit too much can cause a paradoxical effect evident in an increase in oily skin and acne.

Diet and Nutrition Pillar Principles to Treat PMS

- **Diet recommendations**. Many of the women who suffer from PMS have significant nutritional deficiencies. Before recommending any vitamin or mineral supplement, I always encourage patients to rethink their primary nutrient delivery system—the foods they eat every day. The Natural Superwoman diet focuses on consuming whole foods in appropriate portions. In accordance with the PMS diet principles outlined by Dr. Guy E. Abraham, formerly of University of California Los Angeles, in his 1983 article, "Nutritional Factors in the Etiology of the Premenstrual Tension Syndrome," I recommend that women avoid dairy, hydrogenated fat, and "empty calorie" food.

- **Nutritional supplement recommendations**

  Magnesium versus calcium. One of the core principles of my program for treating PMS focuses on replacing all calcium supplements with magnesium supplements. Magnesium provides women with bone support benefits and additionally helps alleviate PMS symptoms. Follow-up studies have confirmed that supplementing absorbable magnesium benefits women who experience PMS symptoms. Note that the nonabsorbable form of magnesium, magnesium oxide, recommended for the treatment of constipation, is a different supplement that will not resolve PMS symptoms. I recommend taking 200 to 1,000 mg, twice a day, with food. Begin with the minimal dose and build up slowly over the course of several weeks. If your dose is too high, you may experience soft stool or a feeling of being too relaxed.

  Vitamin B_6 (pyridoxine). Large doses of vitamin B_6 have been shown to be extremely helpful in alleviating PMS symptoms. Even in very small doses B_6 provides moderate benefits. I recommend 150 to 300 mg, taken daily, with food. Vitamin B_6 should always be taken with 50 mg of B complex.

For mild cases of PMS, simply modifying diet and supplements as described above will help alleviate symptoms within three to six months.

- **Mind and Mood Pillar Principles to decrease PMS.** For more pronounced cases of PMS, adding the nutritional supplements recommended in the mind and mood section to the supplements recommended above will provide greater relief of your mood symptoms.

ACTIVITY MAINTENANCE PILLAR PRINCIPLES
TO DECREASE PMS

If you've noticed that going for a run or visiting the gym for an hour seems to resolve your PMS symptoms, you're not alone. Studies indicate that physical activity can relieve many of the discomforts of PMS.

Treating Fertility Challenges with Progesterone

You cannot enjoy optimal fertility without a normalized progesterone level. In my practice, I use bioidentical progesterone in capsules and sublingual drops to balance progesterone levels and increase fertility. I believe that capsules and drops are the optimal delivery mechanisms to increase your levels of this hormone. Unfortunately, most physicians who specialize in promoting fertility and who use progesterone as part of their treatment program, use two forms of progesterone therapy that I find less effective:

- Oil-based injectable progesterone, an effective but painful remedy. Or:
- Crinone, a bioidentical progesterone available in vaginal cream or suppository form that is available by perscription. My concern about this product is that it contains hydrogenated oil, a harmful trans fat. I object to the use of these fats vaginally, just as I would object to their general consumption. But more important, the problem with using this product or *any* vaginal form of progesterone to promote fertility is that its vaginal application

alarmingly causes the lining of the uterus to thin, resulting in a *lower rate* of embryonic implantation.

Treating Irregular Periods with Progesterone

If you have irregular periods, do not agree to take birth control pills, regardless of your age. Not only will it not remedy the problem of irregular periods, it may even aggravate the condition.

Why is this? Low or no progesterone production is the most common reason for women's irregular periods. The birth control pill prevents conception by suppressing and effectively shutting down the system that causes women to ovulate and produce progesterone. Instead, the pill provides two chemicals—neither capable of replacing all of the functions of your own natural estrogen and progesterone—and produces an artificial menstrual cycle, but does not correct the progesterone deficiency that caused the irregular periods in the first place. In many ways, the birth control pill aggravates the condition.

Before beginning any treatment for irregular periods, ask your physician to rule out pregnancy, thyroid deficiency, pathology in the uterus, and perimenopause Bioidentical progesterone in capsule or cream form can be an excellent treatment tool to maintain your rhythmic menstrual cycle.

A WARNING AGAINST INJECTABLE PROVERA AS A METHOD OF BIRTH CONTROL

In addition to all of the significant side effects associated with the chemical medication Provera, there are other specific problems in using injectable Provera, known as Depo-Provera (medroxyprogesterone acetate), as a method of birth control often recommended to young women, including:

(continued)

It takes years for a woman to resume her normal menstrual cycle after concluding her Depo-Provera treatment.

Appreciable weight gain.

Increase in incidence of urinary tract infections (UTIs).

Increase in the incidence of diabetes.

Increase in risk of chlamydia and gonorrhea infection.

Increase in rate of acquisition of HIV infection, meaning, women on Depo-Provera are more likely to become infected with HIV.

Increase in rate of outward infection, meaning women on Depo-Provera increase their ability to infect others with HIV by increasing the "shedding" of the HIV virus.

Moreover, in studies on primates infected with the primate version of HIV, known as SHIV, treatment with Depo-Provera suppresses their cellular immunity, further compromising an already-compromised immunity. In the face of this evidence, would you subject your body—or your daughter's—to this medication?

In reading about the many benefits of optimizing progesterone levels using bioidentical progesterone, do you wonder why you don't use it? Alternatively, if you are one of the many women currently taking one of the chemical medications that claim to provide you with the safe benefits of progesterone, I encourage you to reconsider your current course of treatment.

6 • Human Growth Hormone: The Misunderstood Partner

QUICK QUIZ

Answer the following questions designed to assess whether you might be experiencing deficiency in human growth hormone (HGH):

Do you feel fatigued?

Do you find that you must sleep more than eight hours, and when you do, you still feel tired?

Have you lost your sense of confidence?

Do you feel more insecure than in the past?

Do you feel that something may go wrong with your plans?

Do you require more approval and reassurance than usual?

Have you lost interest in new projects?

Are you not interested in trying new things?

Are you anxious? Does this affect your quality of sleep?

(continued)

Do you find that jet lag has a worse than usual effect on you?

Do you find that you have more colds and bouts of the flu than usual?

Do you find that you heal more slowly?

Do you gain fat in your midsection and chest?

Do your face, eyes, and cheeks look droopy?

Do you think you have more wrinkles than this time last year?

Do your lips look thinner?

Does the flesh on the underside of your arms sag?

Do you find that your muscles don't respond as well to exercise?

As is not the case with a deficiency of estrogen or progesterone, where certain symptoms evidence a clear need to optimize your hormones, the symptoms of HGH deficiency are not so clear-cut. If you identify with any of these questions, then you may wish to explore the possibility that your body may be producing suboptimal levels of HGH. The sections that follow address some of the reasons you may benefit from optimizing your levels.

HUMAN GROWTH HORMONE BASICS

Human growth hormone (HGH) is produced by the pituitary gland and reaches peak production around age sixteen. The normal range is between 180 and 780. However, when your HGH level is tested, your blood is not tested for HGH itself. Instead, you are tested for a substance called insulin-like growth factor 1 (IGF-1), which is produced by the liver at the prompting of HGH. Taller, more muscular people have a significantly higher level of IGF-1, and shorter, less muscular people have a naturally lower level of IGF-1.

The taller and more muscular you are, the higher your optimal peak HGH production is expected to be. The shorter you are and the less muscle mass you have, the lower your peak HGH production is expected to be. By the age of fifty, humans lose 50 percent of their normal HGH production.

However, because of the way scientists learned about this hormone, the very idea of a normal range is misleading. As is the case in other areas of medicine, normal was not established by testing healthy young adults; instead, scientists used the blood taken from two extreme ends of the population that came in for human growth hormone testing—the very short and the very tall. This means that the average woman cannot simply rely on news that her HGH blood levels are within normal range.

More disturbing is that HGH levels seem to be generally declining. In my practice I currently observe significantly lower levels of blood HGH than I saw fifteen years ago. I often see young women with the same levels as their much older mothers, even though the two women share the same height and muscle profile. While scientists have not yet addressed and explored why this is happening, the results are that younger and younger women are experiencing the symptoms described in the Quick Quiz at the start of this section—more prevalent cold and flu, slower healing, fat in their midsection, droopy skin and flesh, thinner lips, and less responsive muscle—all symptoms generally associated with much older women.

In other words, the idea of what normal is must be reconceived on an optimal and individual basis.

Many patients who come to speak to me about HGH therapy first discuss their concern that supplementing HGH will cause them to develop cancerous tumors. I'm perplexed by these fears because, currently, the FDA approves HGH treatment for three groups:

- Relatively small children who want to grow in height.
- Emaciated AIDS patients.
- Older adults who have lost most of their ability to produce growth hormone, a condition called Adult Growth Hormone Deficiency syndrome.

In all three of these cases, the treatment groups—young children, AIDS patients, and the elderly—are very vulnerable, and their treatment doses are sky-high relative to those discussed in this section. The scientific world has never reported an increased incidence of cancer in these groups. Despite this, women who may choose to avail themselves of relatively minute amounts of HGH are bombarded by mainstream media warnings of cancer and other disastrous consequences. As a medical professional, I am perplexed by this.

In this chapter, my aim is to clear the controversy and emphasize the safety of responsible HGH use, while presenting you with scientific evidence to substantiate the safe benefits of HGH treatment.

BENEFITS OF HGH

- **Protects against cardiovascular disease.** HGH treatment significantly protects against cardiovascular disease in the following ways:

  - HGH treatment decreases cholesterol, triglycerides, and fibrinogen levels. Studies have found that increased levels of these three elements increase the incidence of cardiovascular disease.
  - HGH prevents and slows progression of arterial sclerosis, the blockage of arteries that increases the incidence of cardiovascular disease.
  - HGH significantly improves the condition of women with chronic heart failure. Studies have found that women at the "end stage" of heart disease actually improve their condition when they use growth hormone.

  However, my feeling is, we need not wait until our heart is failing in order to begin enjoying the benefits of HGH on our cardiovascular system.

- **Bone support.** In general, studies indicate that treatment with HGH improves bone density by 1 percent per year. One way it does this is by improving amylin levels, a hormone that increases bone density. Specifically, treatment with HGH improves bone density in hips and growth of bone in the spine.

In my clinical experience, the only patients in whom I did not observe HGH to have a bone-building effect is those women who failed to consume adequate amounts of protein in connection with eating disorders that include anorexia nervosa. As a physician, I am happy to have a tool that builds bone, as most of the osteoporosis medications available to women simply stop the process of bone loss. For this reason, I am enthusiastic about recommending HGH treatment as part of a bone-building program, where HGH is taken in normal, low doses. In fact, one patient reported that since beginning her HGH treatment, she has grown two inches! As a five-foot-three adult male, I wish this would happen to me!

HGH AND NATURAL SUPERWOMAN EATING

For more information on how your natural HGH production can work in concert with Natural Superwoman eating to minimize markers of aging, see Chapter 1, on the diet and nutrition pillar.

- **Body fat.** HGH is an incredible fat burner. In fact, it targets fat that is the hardest to burn—the omental, trunk, or visceral fat that surrounds internal organs and collects in the midsection. While it's true that HGH's fat-burning efforts yield better results in men than women, when women supplement low doses of growth hormone, as recommended in the sections that follow, they also lose body fat. One of the reasons that HGH burns fat is that it increases adiponectin, a hormone that breaks up fat. In fact, children with low levels of HGH also have very low levels of adiponectin.

HGH also improves your capacity to exercise. When young adults exercise, their natural HGH level rises. When older adults exercise, there is no increase in HGH levels. As a medical professional, I regularly consult women who wish to maintain the level of fitness they have naturally enjoyed their whole lives. It seems logical that they may wish to turn to HGH treatment to maintain their natural, physiologically appropriate activity level, though I strongly condemn the use of HGH treatment for the purpose of bodybuilding-type muscle development.

HGH BENEFITS THE MIND AND MOOD PILLAR

- **Improves sleep.** HGH production naturally peaks between midnight to one a.m. and has a significant effect on sleep. Studies indicate that women with low HGH levels do not sleep well and treatment with HGH helps women sleep. One of the ways in which HGH helps is by reducing cortisol. High levels of nighttime cortisol cause women to experience insomnia and feel anxious and wired. On the other hand, women with lower levels of HGH often feel sleepy throughout the day and fail to wake up feeling rested. HGH treatment helps these women fall asleep at night, experience better quality sleep, and feel more alert throughout the day. Although general HGH doses are taken during the day, for women who have trouble sleeping, I recommend that they take HGH thirty to sixty minutes before bedtime. Rarely, treatment with HGH at bedtime results in a paradoxical effect—making you feel more awake at bedtime. If this occurs, simply take your dose during the day, rather than at night.

- **Improves motivation and feeling of well-being.** HGH has a positive effect on mood. When adults receive HGH treatment with low, physiological doses, they report a feeling of well-being and confidence. From these men and women, I often hear the following:

"I'm back."

"Life is worth living"

"I feel self-confident again."

"I'm painting again."

"I've begun a new project"

"I've gone back to school."

• **Improves mental function.** Studies indicate that HGH improves mental performance and memory. Higher levels of HGH are also associated with a faster and more effective recovery time for adults who have suffered a stroke. In addition, in my practice I have observed that HGH treatment also restores overall mental motivation, an interest in tackling new information, and the sharing of information with others—all characteristics associated with a "young mind," rather than an older, more close-minded mental attitude. Although this may seem like something more properly attributed to general increased body energy, a big part of feeling this way is governed by mental function related to attitude; HGH has a direct effect in improving attitude.

HGH BENEFITS TO OTHER HORMONES

• **Promoting efficacy of other hormones.** Contrary to what some people believe, supplementing HGH *does not* decrease your own body's production of HGH. In fact, studies indicate that HGH improves ovarian hormone production in general. Because HGH improves hormone function, it may also increase your production of testoterone, causing oily skin and a more physically aggressive attitude. If this resonates with your experience and you supplement testosterone, reduce your dosage of testosterone. HGH may also decrease your production of cortisol. If your adrenal function is normal, this will simply allow you to manage stress in a more calm way. However, if you are not producing enough cortisol due to adrenal deficiency, further reducing your cortisol with HGH is not ideal. For this reason, it is imperative to establish proper adrenal function before beginning HGH treatment. Finally, HGH also improves thyroid function. I have found that HGH improves the production of T4 and the conversion of T4 to T3, the most active thyroid hormone. When this occurs, women with untreated thyroid deficiency will find that their condition will improve, and those who supplement thyroid may have to decrease their dose.

- **Fertility.** HGH promotes fertility in a number of key ways. Specifically, HGH participates in ovarian follicle development, improves women's response to Clomid, the oral fertility treatment, and in vitro fertilization (IVF). In light of the great expense and effort associated with Clomid and IVF treatments, my feeling is that anything that safely improves their efficacy is an important option for women to know about.

  In my practice, I see many women for whom conventional fertility treatments are not helpful. I continue to be amazed when I observe how HGH and other hormone and nutritional supplements improve fertility success.

OTHER CONDITIONS TREATABLE WITH HGH

- **Fibromyalgia.** Women with fibromyalgia enjoy increased energy with HGH treatment.

- **Anemia.** HGH treatment should always be considered for women with anemia.

- **Skin function.** HGH significantly benefits the overall skin function, including improving elasticity and rate of healing, while decreasing the incidence and severity of scarring. I have noticed that more and more plastic surgeons are prescribing HGH before and after surgery, and it has been my personal observation that when women are treated with HGH prior to elective cosmetic surgery, they enjoy less bruising and swelling and overall faster rates of healing. In addition, studies indicate that burn victims treated with HGH have a far lower mortality rate than those not treated with HGH.

- **Hair loss and growth.** In my practice, I have observed that HGH reduces head hair loss, and promotes the growth of head hair, without increasing the growth of body hair.

HOW TO SUPPLEMENT HGH

More and more, I meet new patients who have already put themselves on an HGH treatment program by buying it over the Internet or by obtaining it through other means. This concerns me, because HGH treatment requires proper history, exam, and blood workup, in addition to the individualized dose recommended and follow-up in order to prevent interference with the function of other hormones. For example, this treatment is currently not appropriate for patients in active cancer treatment, nor is it appropriate for those with untreated decreased adrenal function.

After taking the patient's appropriate history and physical exam, I recommend the following baseline blood tests:

- Lipids (cholesterol series)
- C-reactive protein (CRP)
- Thyroid function test (TFT)
- Insulin
- Hemoglobin A1C
- Glucose
- Complete blood count (CBC)
- Testosterone
- Cortisol
- Insulin-like growth factor 1 (IGF-1)
- Insulin-like growth factor binding protein 3 (IGFBP-3)

Setting your dose. The doses described here are a small fraction of those recommended in reports on safe HGH use. HGH is supplemented by injection transdermally, or just under the skin. When recommending that patients consider HGH treatment, I suggest that they begin with 0.5 to 1.5 mg weekly, and the maximum dose, 3 mg, weekly. I generally recommend that women take HGH during the day and before physical activity, unless it is taken to promote sleep, in which case it should be taken thirty to sixty minutes before bedtime.

HGH treatment must be accompanied by constant follow-up by a physician who has experience in low-dose HGH therapy.

Nicole's Story

Nicole, thirty-four, is a five-foot-eight-inch, 125-pound personal trainer. In the last few years, she has complained of multiple injuries and poor healing. She also reports that she has mental fatigue, requires a lot more sleep than she used to, and never feels rested. When she does lay her head down at night, she finds that she cannot easily fall asleep, despite having spent an entire day feeling tired. Her diet is ideal and she exercises two hours a day. Despite this, she told me that she's accumulated four pounds of belly fat that she cannot seem to get rid of. Her blood workup was relatively normal, besides two relative abnormalities—her night-time saliva cortisol levels were higher than her afternoon levels, and, her the level of insulin-like growth factor 1 (the marker used to measure natural HGH levels), though still within normal limits, was significantly lower than expected for her age. This last blood reading was consistent with my observation of seeing lower and lower HGH levels in younger women, and that concerned me. In response to this, I recommended that she take 1.33 mg weekly, divided into daily morning doses. She returned to my office after three months and reported enjoying great daytime energy and no longer needing to take naps and also sleeping well at night. Moreover, the belly fat that she couldn't lose was long gone.

POSSIBLE SIDE EFFECTS

If you faithfully follow the guidelines above, side effects associated with HGH treatment are mild, easily recognizable, and simply resolved.

- **Water retention,** the most common side effect, expresses itself with swelling of the hands and feet. You may find that you have a hard time removing your rings. In the many years I have worked with this hormone, only once have I seen a patient with significant swelling in both hands. A 25 percent reduction of your dose should resolve this effect within one week. Unlike the recommendations I make for other hormones, I strongly condemn any attempt to resolve this side effect with the use of diuretics in place of dose reduction.

- **Carpal tunnel syndrome,** a pain, swelling, or loss of sensation in the median nerve of the wrist, while very rare in low doses, is nonetheless the second-most common side effect associated with HGH treatment. It may occur if you experience water retention in your hands and wrists. If you find that you experience wrist pain, simply reduce your dose by 25 percent and the condition should resolve within one week.

- **Joint pain** may occur within a few weeks of initial use in approximately 10 percent of patients, but rarely appears beyond this period of time. A reduction of your dose by 25 to 50 percent will resolve your discomfort within one week. In my long experience prescribing this hormone, I have only seen one patient who was unable to resolve her joint pain at any lower dose, and obviously this one woman was not a candidate for HGH treatment.

- **Agitation** and a feeling of being hyper is an incredibly rare side effect, and is easily resolved with a decrease of your dose by 25 percent.

- **Increase of white and red blood cells.** HGH increases your red and white blood cell count. Always monitor this increase with your physician's assistance to insure that it does not surpass levels that you and your doctor are comfortable with.

- **Unreported side effects.** In the twelve years I have treated patients with HGH, I have seen only three women who developed a small growth of fat tissue on the site of the HGH injection, documented by imaging (X-ray and ultrasound). Usually, HGH melts fat wherever it is injected. In my clinical follow-up with these women, I discovered that they were injecting their HGH into the same area over and over again, rather than alternating injection sites with every dose. In these rare cases, simply ceasing to inject at the affected site and rotating injection sites resolved this condition within three to six months.

DOES HGH CAUSE CANCER?

This section presents the most current scientific and clinical information that will enable you to make a decision about how *you* feel about HGH treatment out of informed reason, rather than out of fear.

If you take cancer cells in a petri dish and add HGH, the cancer cells will grow. However, while petri dish studies can be helpful in establishing smaller medical processes, the human body is not a petri dish—our bodies are significantly more complicated and have many more checks and balances. One chief difference between a human body and a petri dish is that our bodies have robust immune systems designed to target and protect against the development and growth of cancer cells. In fact, in studies on actual human beings, HGH has been shown to support and reinforce the immune system.

- Increasing monocyst, an important part of the white cell defense
- Increasing glutathione, a key antioxidant, and decreasing nuclear factor-kappa beta, a toxic pro-inflammatory

- Increasing natural killer-cell (NK cell) activity, one of the body's chief anticancer programs; studies on mice afflicted with stomach cancer treated with HGH indicate that HGH prevents the accelerated tumor growth
- Increasing insulin-like growth factor binding protein 3 (IGFBP3), a substance known for decreasing the incidence of breast cancer
- Increasing erythropoietin (EPO) secretion, which builds red cells
- Building cancer-fighting white cells and lymphocytes
- Increasing adiponectin, which prevents the development of cancer by inhibiting angiogenesis, the formation of new blood vessels by the cancer cells
- Reversing bone marrow deterioration associated with aging

HGH builds, maintains, and prevents the decline of the very system that protects us against cancer. If the dish experts would add all of the complex components of our immune system enhanced by HGH to each petri dish, they would have seen very different results. Once one understands the difference between a petri dish and studies on real women, men, and even children, it becomes obvious why studies on adults and children treated with HGH show no evidence of an increase in cancer rates.

The Growth Hormone Research Society, an organization charged with supervising all FDA-indicated HGH treatments that regularly utilize doses that are two to forty times higher than the doses indicated for the treatment protocol described in the following sections, concluded their 2001 findings summary thus: "The extensive data to date collected on large numbers of children and adults treated with growth hormone indicates that for the current approved indications growth hormone is safe." Of course, in reading the phrase "current approved indications" one would think that means that HGH is not safe for nonindicated treatment; however, the opposite is true. As discussed at the beginning of this chapter, the patients who are given FDA-indicated HGH treatments are the weakest and most vulnerable patient groups—they include children, AIDS patients, and fragile elderly adults. These three groups are treated with two to fourteen times the maximum dose and four to forty-two times the minimum dose described in the treatment outlined in the following sections.

In other words, mainstream science has concluded that even in instances where HGH treatment is administered in very large doses to the most vulnerable members of our population, HGH is both FDA-approved and safe. As a medical professional, my conclusion from all the studies cited above is that giving a fraction of these doses to far healthier adults is only that much safer. And to the extent that patients have concerns about colon cancer, routine and thorough colonoscopies—testing that is far superior to mammograms—will provide a measure of assurance.

DOES HGH CAUSE DIABETES?

Just as women are erroneously warned about a connection between HGH and cancer, there is also an unfounded concern that links HGH and diabetes. In the twelve years I have personally used HGH and recommended it to my indicated-patient population, using a dose of 1 to 3 mg a week, I have yet to see a single follow-up test result indicate diabetes, prediabetes, or even sugar-metabolism deterioration. On the contrary, I have generally observed an improvement. In studies where HGH treatment was administered to diabetic, obese patients with very poor sugar control, this group improved its insulin sensitivity, lost weight, improved cholesterol and triglyceride levels, and lowered blood sugar levels.

How can HGH improve diabetes? Likely, HGH:

- Increases amlin, a hormone recently approved to treat diabetes.
- Increases adiponectin, a substance that protects against diabetes.
- Reduces overall body fat, and therefore contributes to reversing the many destructive conditions associated with diabetes.

Very low dosages of HGH protect against, rather than cause, diabetes.

7 • DHEA:
The Master Hormone

Unlike other hormones discussed in this book, DHEA does not lend itself to a quick listing of symptoms that can be incorporated into a quiz. This is because the function of DHEA touches on so many other hormones.

Eva's Story

Eva, thirty-nine, came to visit me for an early evening appointment, apologizing for seeming a bit on edge. She'd put her husband in charge of picking up and feeding the kids, and she just knew the house would be a whirlwind of evening cleanup when she finally made it home after this office visit and a long day of work. She looked tired, but more so, she looked overwhelmed. When we spoke, she confirmed that she was experiencing extreme stress, was overworked, and didn't think that she ever had enough time for herself, her husband, or her two kids. She felt she was doing everything badly and was disappointed in herself for still carrying around those last fifteen pounds left over from pregnancy. While she was happy to make lifestyle changes (i.e., diet and

(continued)

exercise), she said that she knows herself, and that she would ultimately not keep up with a program that required her to take a fistful of pills every day. She joked that she could probably handle taking one pill, like a multivitamin.

Her medical history revealed that her father had died of heart disease at a young age, and that her mother was currently battling breast cancer. In evaluating her blood, I found that her hemoglobin A1c level evidenced that she was prediabetic. Her overall cholesterol was normal, but she had low HDL ("good" cholesterol) and high triglycerides. She confirmed that between work lunches and meals with her kids, she tended to eat a high-carbohydrate diet. Eva's morning cortisol was on the higher level of normal and her DHEA was extremely low at 54 ug/dL.

With so many benefits associated with ideal levels of DHEA, in general, I felt that every aspect of Eva's health—and of your health—can be improved and protected by supplementing this vital hormone. None of us can escape the conditions that DHEA protects us from, so I think that supplementing DHEA on an individualized basis is as natural as DHEA itself.

This is particularly salient when you consider that DHEA levels drop during a woman's life. Women's DHEA levels peak between the ages of twenty and thirty, and plummet by 70 percent between ages fifty to sixty. The scientific community explains that DHEA levels decline less after this age. After hysterectomy, doctors are able to track a measurable decline in DHEA production as soon as one week following the procedure. In my clinical experience, I observe a much earlier and more significant drop, which I attribute to significant stress and the use of oral contraceptives, and a more consistent decline as women age.

I immediately spoke with Eva about lifestyle changes based on the other three pillars, introducing her to the lower, more favorable carbohydrate principles and to caloric reduction consistent with Natural Superwoman eating, and the stress-relieving steps of the mind and mood pillar. I encouraged her to increase her choice of physical activity per the activity maintenance pillar.

When it came to discussing nutrients and, separately, the hormone balance pillar, Eva requested that I limit my recommendations to one supplement: I told Eva to take DHEA.

In this section, you'll learn more about why a woman like Eva is the ideal candidate to supplement DHEA. In general, with her family history of heart disease on her father's side and breast cancer on her mother's, she requires DHEA to work in concert with her other hormones to protect against these two serious threats to women's health. DHEA will also be helpful to her other current conditions: it serves as a significant stress releaser, improves insulin sensitivity, and slows down and begins to reverse a prediabetic course. DHEA will also energize Eva and help her lose belly fat, in addition to helping her enjoy a better response to physical activity. Finally, DHEA will provide an overall improvement of her sense of well-being.

Eva began taking 5 mg with her breakfast, so that she could take her supplement one time a day when she was at home. She increased her dose by 5 mg every two or three weeks and settled on a final dose of 15 mg per day, because she began to feel edgy when she increased her dosage to 20 mg. Her own body alerted her to its optimal dose.

Eva came back to the office four months later and reported that she had been relatively loyal to her diet and activity goals, she was breathing better, but had a longer path to reduce her stress. She had an improved sense of well-being, lost seven pounds, and now had more time to do the things she liked or needed to do. She was less likely to lose her temper with the kids and had more time and energy to share with her husband. Her blood work revealed that her DHEA was up to 210 ug/dL. Her HDL, or "good" cholesterol, went up, and her triglycerides decreased. Her hemoglobin A1c dropped from 6 to 5.6. She enjoyed less belly fat and slightly more muscle definition. Overall, her outlook on all the things on her plate seemed far more manageable, and she joked that DHEA seemed to add sleeping and waking hours to the clock. Could that be?

Obviously, literally, it cannot. But in terms of offering the ability to achieve daily goals for many women, DHEA is a lifesaver.

DHEA gets a great deal of attention in mainstream news. As usual, in the aggregate, the news is confusing—some reports are fascinating and promising, and others are controversial and negative, claiming that DHEA produces side effects while providing no concrete benefits. As explained, DHEA is not a cut-and-dried hormone, so it makes sense that its benefits may not lend themselves to easy news sound bites. I've treated more than 7,000 women with DHEA in the last fifteen years. Currently, at least a thousand of my active patients use DHEA. My point in sharing this with you is simply to clarify that my advice on DHEA is not based on the theoretical analysis of articles on the subject, but rather from the perspective of a health-care provider who sees women who supplement DHEA every day, and who sees how it affects their lives.

The aim here is to share with you what DHEA does in your body, why additional amounts are so beneficial, why there is controversy about this hormone, and why, despite this controversy, DHEA continues to be a safe natural supplement, and, finally, why you may wish to add DHEA to your natural supplement program.

DHEA BASICS

DHEA is the body's most abundant hormone, the majority of which is produced by the adrenal gland and a small portion in the ovaries. Most DHEA found in your body is bound to a sulfate molecule called DHEA-sulfate (DHEAS), which renders it inactive, though it is ready to be used when you need it.

Although many people think of DHEA as a male hormone, or androgen, women actually produce at least two-thirds of the amount of DHEA produced by men. This indicates that androgens play an important role in women's hormonal health, a role that has been completely underestimated by the scientific community to date.

HOW DHEA BENEFITS
THE NATURAL SUPERWOMAN

DHEA provides you with significant benefits in a whole range of health concerns. Specifically:

- **DHEA protects against breast cancer.** In the chapter on breast cancer we describe the benefits of DHEA on this devastating disease. Studies confirm these benefits:

  - Supplementing DHEA decreases incidence of breast cancer.
  - When human breast cancer cells were introduced into the body of mice, supplementing the mice with DHEA suppressed the growth of the breast cancer cells.
  - DHEA generally inhibits the progression of breast cancer.

  In fact, the most prestigious endocrine journal, *Endocrine Reviews,* published a thirty-page article, with 336 references, by Dr. Fernando La Brie in Quebec, explaining how androgens like DHEA and testosterone protect women from breast cancer.

  Why is this? One of the most common breast cancer treatments available today is a group of medications called aromatase inhibitors. In the absence of androgens like DHEA and testosterone, these medications are not as efficient as they could be. DHEA suppresses the production of 4-hydroxy estrone, a metabolite of estrogen that is understood to be a major contributor to the development of breast cancer.

  Scientific evidence confirms DHEA as a powerful tool in the prevention, protection, and treatment of breast cancer. The sheer volume of articles published on this subject in established, mainstream medical journals should provide women with comfort that the men and women who devote their lives to understanding how DHEA affects a woman's body believe that DHEA does not cause the development of breast cancer, but rather protects women from it.

- **DHEA protects against other forms of cancer as well.** Multiple studies describe the general anticancerous effect of DHEA. In addition, specific studies on animals indicate the anticancerous effects of DHEA on pancreatic, colon, and prostate cancers.

- **DHEA has been shown to protect against cardiovascular disease.** In the section addressing cardiovascular disease, we discussed how DHEA can help in one of the most serious health concerns confronting women today. Cardiovascular disease affects more women each and every year. Throughout this book, we highlight how estrogen and other nutritional and hormonal tools can protect women from this deadly disease. DHEA directly adds to the benefit provided by estrogen and every other tool that supports the cardiovascular system. Specifically:

  - DHEA inhibits *platelet aggregation,* one of the first signs of a troubled cardiovascular system.
  - DHEA reverses the aging process of the left ventricle of the heart.
  - Young women with polycystic ovarian syndrome (POS) who are prone to cardiovascular disease because of their condition have high DHEA levels; studies have proven that the young women's levels of DHEA are high as a cardioprotective response of their bodies.

In the many years I have spent treating women with DHEA, I have never observed a negative effect on the cardiovascular system.

- **DHEA has been shown to protect against diabetes.** One of the most problematic and growing hazards today is the high frequency of diabetes and insulin resistance. Where previously diabetes was considered a disease of the old, we now regularly observe alarming rates in very young children, young adults, and the greater adult populations. Treatment with DHEA has been shown to improve the overall condition of diabetes. Specifically, DHEA:

  - Improves insulin sensitivity.
  - Increases the pancreatic cells that produce insulin, in studies on rats.
  - Increases insulin production, in studies on rats.
  - Decreases insulin resistance in humans with coronary heart disease.

- **DHEA increases adiponectin, a hormone that decreases fat and cardiovascular disease, and prevents the progression of cancer by decreasing its ability to create new cancer-spreading blood vessels.**

  In simple terms, adiponectin fights what the average American diet—high in saturated fat, carbohydrates, and sugar—does to your body in the short and long term. I mention adiponectin in this section because supplementary DHEA is an easy way to increase your adiponectin levels. However, increasing adiponectin is just one of the reasons that DHEA protects Natural Superwomen from heart disease, cancer, and diabetes. In addition, DHEA provides the following benefits:

- **DHEA enhances immunity and protects against autoimmune disease.** Specifically:

  - Increases natural killer (NK) cell activity, one of the strongest cancer-protective tools available to the body.
  - Slows the onset of autoimmune disease.

- Improves skin wound healing.
- Enhances your body's protection against cold, flu, allergies, viral disease, parasites, and bacteria.
- While protecting you from infectious disease, reduces your body's inflammation response by decreasing pro-inflammatory cytokines, which decreases incidence of colitis, rheumatoid arthritis, lupus, psoriasis, and endometriosis.
- Decreases the incidence of colds, flu, and allergies.
- Reduces osteoarthritis and general joint pain.
- Functions as a general antioxidant, reducing free radicals in the body.

Indeed, many of the women to whom I recommend DHEA report a decrease in colds and flu. When it comes to autoimmune diseases such as arthritis, the benefits of supplementing DHEA require three to six months of taking the highest dose you can tolerate in order to see a difference. But then again, it took years to develop, so a few months to remedy doesn't seem that bad.

DHEA BENEFITS THE MIND AND MOOD PILLAR

As a hormone that can help adjust your adrenal response and improve your general feeling of well-being, DHEA can be a powerful partner in helping you balance your mind and mood.

- **DHEA decreases depression and increases your feeling of well-being.** Studies show that women who supplement DHEA report a decrease in symptoms of depression and an increase in self-confidence and emotional strength.

- **DHEA reduces anxiety.** When used properly, DHEA can be significantly helpful in reducing anxiety. Specifically, DHEA:

- Decreases cortisol.
- Increases estrogen.
- Increases progesterone and allopregnenolone, which in turn increases GABA levels, the neurotransmitter that promotes a feeling of calm.

- **Improves memory.** Specifically, DHEA:

  - Generally protects the hippocampus, the memory center of the brain, from injury and free radicals.
  - Provides an effective treatment in both vascular (vessel) and neuronal (nerve) diseases affecting the brain, including stroke.

In my practice, I have found that the most significant effect of DHEA comes from its ability to moderate and control our stress response. By reducing fight-or-flight instincts that shut down thinking in order to channel energy to outrunning a predator, our capacity for the whole range of cognitive abilities, including memory, increases significantly. For more information on stress management, see Chapter 11.

DHEA BENEFITS THE ACTIVITY MAINTENANCE PILLAR

DHEA plays an important role in supporting your activity-maintenance pillar because it promotes a feeling of well-being, supports your adrenal function, and can be converted into testosterone when needed. This translates into the following benefits:

- **Improves muscle development.** Studies indicate that DHEA improves muscle mass and strength after resistance exercises, and also reverses age-related changes in fat mass. In my practice, I have noted that

DHEA's effect on muscle and fat is individualized—in some women the change is minimal and in others the effect is significant.

- **Improves bone strength.** DHEA plays a significant role in improving bone mass. Treatment for one year has been shown to improve bone density in the spine by building new bone cells and decreasing bone loss. In my practice, I turn to DHEA as a complement to other natural supplements rather than prescribing Fosamax, Boniva, and other medications. Consider supplementing DHEA and the natural bone aids recommended in Chapter 16 when looking for something to assist you in reversing existing bone loss and protecting you from further loss.

- **DHEA is necessary for high-altitude cardiovascular performance.** DHEA is essential for the physiological acclimation that climbers, hikers, and alpine (downhill) skiers must undergo in order to function at high altitudes. Women who do not live at high altitude year-round would greatly benefit from supplementing DHEA when planning and enjoying a high-altitude climb, hike, or ski trip.

- **DHEA affects sexual arousal and response.** A great deal has been written about DHEA and sexuality. Studies on menopausal women who were shown erotic movies with and without a 300 mg megadose of DHEA indicated that DHEA provided a significant increase in mental and physiological sexual arousal, as the women enjoyed increased sex drive and better orgasmic response. The average woman can only tolerate 10 to 15 mg without side effects. For this reason, I don't believe that DHEA is a viable enhancer of sexual arousal and response. However, I have observed that women who supplement DHEA in conventional doses enjoy an increase in arousal and response associated with the general increase of well-being produced by DHEA. In addition, when women apply DHEA vaginally thirty minutes before sex, some enjoy an immediate increase in arousal and the quality of their orgasm and other sexual responses.

DHEA BENEFITS THE HORMONE PILLAR

- **DHEA has a profound effect on the production of hormones in your body.** In essence, it functions like a "master hormone," converting into other hormones when necessary. This characteristic makes it unique and important. Specifically, DHEA:

  - Increases human growth hormone (HGH) and reduces the overall amount of growth hormone required for any given treatment; in my practice, I always prefer to include DHEA in any HGH treatment protocol I recommend.
  - Increases allopregnenolone and endorphins; this explains why supplementing DHEA makes us feel calm.
  - Converts into estrogen.
  - Converts into other androgens, like testosterone, but only in specific cells designed for this conversion; from a clinical perspective, this means that these higher hormone levels may not be detectable in blood tests, since the conversion occurs within cells, rather than in the bloodstream.
  - Increases progesterone levels.
  - Supports the adrenal gland, by reducing cortisol and thereby reducing stress.

  In addition to general hormone production support:

- **DHEA uniquely identifies suboptimal cortisol production.** DHEA serves as a tremendously helpful measuring tool in understanding the level of adrenal stress and function. DHEA levels will be low in the early stages of adrenal overproduction, when cortisol levels are still high, and even lower in the later stages of adrenal exhaustion, when cortisol levels are low. Either way, low DHEA levels serve as telltale signs that attention is needed.

DHEA decreases high levels of cortisol. In women with adrenal deficiency and low cortisol who are fatigued, depressed, and very weak, treatment with DHEA will elevate their mood, energy, and general feeling of well-being by mimicking the beneficial properties of the cortisol that these women lack. In my practice, I find that this group is generally able to tolerate higher levels of DHEA.

- **DHEA can correct defects associated with thyroid diseases.** Two of the most common thyroid-related autoimmune conditions, Graves' disease and Hashimoto's thyroiditis, are attributed to autoimmune defects in the natural killer (NK) cells. DHEA can correct these defects.

- **Miscellaneous hormonal benefits of optimal DHEA levels.** In addition to the specific hormonal effects above, DHEA provides the following hormonal and physiological benefits:

  - Decreases hot flashes, likely because of DHEA's conversion to estrogen.
  - Improves fertility treatment response in women who had been unresponsive prior to supplementing DHEA. In my practice, I recommend a physiological dose to women who wish to conceive.

- **DHEA may be a key to sustainable longevity.** While I wouldn't call DHEA the "fountain of youth," as a physician devoting my professional life to the study of hormones and quality life extension, I can't help but notice a connection between higher levels of DHEA and longer, healthy living. For example, of all the concepts currently under review on the subject of living longer, the one program all medical professionals seem to agree on is the notion that limiting your caloric intake consistently increases life span. This is the core of Natural Superwoman eating. Interestingly, DHEA levels rise with the implementation of the calorie reduction principles of Natural Superwoman eating.

Moreover, in studies on long-lived populations, relative DHEA levels are able to predict rates of death. For example, in a three-year study on 963 adults in their eighties, those with lower DHEA levels were 64 percent more likely to die during the course of the three-year study.

IS DHEA AN ANABOLIC STERIOD?

The benefits of DHEA are well-known and supported by scientific reports from respected medical journals. Despite this, there is an organized, general assault on women's ability to access it. Bioidentical DHEA has been wrongfully mischaracterized as an anabolic steroid. This mislabeling has gone so far as to cause some lawmakers to attempt to outlaw the use of DHEA supplements altogether. For this reason, some women who approach their doctors about DHEA may hear: "That's a stupid thing to do." Or: "You're taking a risk." Or: "You don't need it."

While the choice of supplementing hormones is an individual one, it is my hope that in sharing medical evidence on the benefits of using DHEA you will realize that the only "stupid" thing about using DHEA is the act of closing your mind to studies that report its benefits in both healthy and recovering people, and the only "risk" you take is losing the opportunity to join this growing group of men and women who enjoy its disease-fighting and health-enhancing attributes. With all due respect to my colleagues, I often find that "You don't need it" generally means "I don't know anything about it." I encourage you to connect with a health-care provider who supports your willingness to look beyond cookie-cutter health care and create a program that suits your individual needs.

IF DHEA IS SO GREAT,
WHY IS THERE CONTROVERSY?

Imagine what would happen if a pharmaceutical company created a drug that decreases heart disease, cancer and breast cancer, diabetes, stress, and fat, while improving mood and memory, sexuality, energy, bone strength and muscle development, and the physiological function of other hormones produced by your body. I'm certain this medication would be fortified in your bread and orange juice, sprayed over your home, added to your water, and included in any other delivery mechanism available.

Medical studies have repeatedly established the far-ranging benefits of DHEA, so why is there still misunderstanding and controversy surrounding this hormone?

In my opinion, controversy regarding DHEA exists for the following reasons:

- **Most doses recommended are far too high.** Most of the studies on DHEA and women are based on dosing that is too high, or supraphysiological doses. Most studies give women 25 to 100 mg daily, some studies call for 1,000 mg daily. In my experience treating more than 7,000 women with DHEA, I have only come across a handful who were able to tolerate more than 50 mg daily. About 10 to 15 percent of women are only able to tolerate 5 mg daily. The average adult can tolerate 10 to 15 mg a day without experiencing side effects. Nonetheless, the very fact that scientists are willing to use such large doses on human studies further supports evidence of its safety.

- **The "normal range" is not consistently defined.** The range of DHEA levels regarded as normal varies by lab. And each one will modify this range from time to time, so that normal results from blood taken from one year to the next may not be consistent. Additionally, the definition of "normal range" is determined by comparing your blood to that of others in your age group, rather than to the blood of healthy young people, which should be the marker for optimal levels. The result is that if you are forty and supplementing DHEA, your lab results may warn you that your DHEA levels are too high, when in fact, the blood levels of your age peers are too low to be of any use to them.

- **Interpretation of tests on DHEA blood levels in women, specifically, is misleading.** Nearly 25 percent of the female population develops a condition called polycystic ovarian syndrome. These women suffer from obesity, a tendency toward diabetes, eating disorders, cardiovascular disease, decreased sex drive, irregular periods, depression, anxiety, and uterine cancer. This group of women is also known to have a relatively high level of DHEA. Scary correlation, right? But studies have proven that this high level of DHEA is their bodies' adaptive and protective mechanism to the onslaught of tendencies associated with polycystic ovarian syndrome. In other words, their bodies respond to their risk of further illness by producing higher levels of DHEA to protect them. Pretty great, isn't it?

  Still, in order to avoid tainted results, these women that science has established as producing higher levels to protect them must be removed from the study group.

  For this reason, I did not include studies on DHEA blood levels. I believe that because of this high predisposition toward polycystic ovarian syndrome, tests based specifically on DHEA blood levels in women are misleading.

- **Many of the studies on DHEA are too short to be meaningful.** Studies on DHEA are commonly three months or shorter in duration. Some last only weeks. Because of the way DHEA expresses itself, studies must be at least six to twelve months in duration in order to be helpful.

- **Studies on DHEA in women are often "blind," but in a bad way.** In many of the studies on DHEA, the named authors never treat or otherwise interact with the women who participate in the studies they publish. Often authors simply review data or questionnaires. Supplementing hormones is so individual and requires a more comprehensive, personal dialogue. My conclusions on how and why DHEA works is based on a multidecade treatment program that involves meeting each woman, listening to her concerns, checking her blood levels, recommending an individual program, and then listening to her personal experience with this program in order to adjust it for maximum benefits. In my experience, this is the only way to treat something as nuanced and complex as the hormonal system, and is therefore the only acceptable means of understanding how supplementing DHEA affects you.

  How can I trust a study reporting that seventeen women were given 50 mg of DHEA for six months with an "absence of side effects"? As mentioned, in my treatment of thousands of women I am not aware of ten women who would tolerate 50 mg without developing acne, head hair loss, and facial hair growth. In my experience, most women given 25 mg, half the dose indicated by this study, would develop severe acne within four weeks and chin hair growth and head hair loss within three months.

  Who are the medical professionals overseeing these studies? What side effects are their questionnaires asking for? Is anyone actually speaking to and seeing the women who participate in these studies?

- **Scare Tactics 101: How to design a medical study that scares people out of using an available remedy.** The majority of studies on treatment of liver cancer with DHEA show that DHEA reduces proliferation of the disease. Yet in articles by opponents of DHEA use, authors routinely cite one study where treatment with DHEA was shown to cause liver cancer. How could this be? Let's look at this study and see how it was conducted.

In the study, mice were given a dose of DHEA that is the human dose equivalent of more than 9,000 mg. Remember, a human adult can only tolerate 10 to 15 mg without experiencing side effects. This dose was administered to these poor mice for more than a year and a half of real time, which is the human equivalent of close to seventy-five years.

It took this much DHEA administered for this long to show that, ultimately, liver function was overwhelmed and the organ developed cancer. In my view, the conclusion of this study should be that DHEA is actually safer than water.

SUPPLEMENTING DHEA

My decision to recommend DHEA treatment to a patient is individualized and based on what a woman reports she feels and what testing reveals.

Unlike with some hormones such as thyroid, estrogen, progesterone, testosterone, and human growth hormone, there are no typical signs of DHEA deficiency. The only symptom that DHEA deficiency shares with testosterone deficiency (although not with any other hormone deficiency) is a loss of body hair, pubic hair, and axillary (underarm) hair.

- **Measuring DHEA blood levels.** In my practice, I do not measure DHEA levels in saliva or urine. The urine test requires collecting urine in a container for twenty-four hours. I find this inconvenient and impractical for my patients; who wants to carry around a canister of urine all day? And, although saliva tests may be helpful in establishing a baseline before beginning DHEA treatment, once treatment has begun, these tests yield results that are so high, they are meaningless to patient follow-up.

Alternatively, in blood tests I measure DHEA-sulfate (DHEAS), rather than DHEA levels, as it provides more stable results. A healthy DHEAS level for a twenty-year-old woman is 50 to 300 ug/dL or 500 to 3,000 ng/ml. I consider a DHEAS level under 150 ug/dL or under 1,000 ng/ml very low in women under age twenty.

Remember, by ages fifty to sixty, most of us have lost 70 percent of the DHEAS level we enjoyed in our twenties, when levels were at their peak. I recommend that patients replace the amount of DHEA that their bodies will tolerate—your own body's tolerance level dictates what it requires.

- **How and when to supplement.** DHEA comes in many forms: capsules, drops, and cream or gels. I don't recommend the cream or gel version, because I find that it has a minimal systemic absorption; to achieve a minimal increase in DHEA blood levels, a patient must use so much that it makes this treatment too expensive.

I recommend drops occasionally, but find them less than ideal because they cause patients' DHEA blood levels to peak too soon and then dissipate quickly.

DHEA capsules are most convenient. They cause DHEA blood levels to reach their peak in three to six hours, and their average levels in eight to twelve hours.

When choosing your DHEA supplement, look for products that are 100 percent pure and micronized, or highly refined. The micronized form diminishes the conversion of DHEA to testosterone, allowing you to use more without experiencing side effects associated with testosterone, including oily skin and breakouts. If you find "bargain" DHEA, consider that the quality may be reduced along with the price—and it may not be a deal at all.

I have seen patients who use a variety of over-the-counter products; some of these women enjoy little or no appreciable rise of DHEAS levels or its benefits. Consider sourcing your supplement from a compounding pharmacy or your physician.

DHEA should be taken in anticipation of the time you want to feel alert, which generally means that you should take it during the day, unless your schedule requires you to feel alert at night.

- **Setting your dose.** I usually recommend that patients begin by taking 5 mg with breakfast or lunch. For a few women, even this low dose will be too much, and they will begin to experience the side effects described below. If this occurs, I recommend reducing the dose to 1 mg with meals. DHEA should always be taken with food. If you take more than 5 mg, you can split this dose between breakfast and lunch. I recommend that patients increase their dose slowly, staying at the same level for at least two weeks. This is because DHEA assists in so many physiological processes that increasing your dose too quickly means that you will not be able to fully appreciate all of the ways it may be helping you.

  Most women can tolerate 10 to 15 mg. Some women may be able to tolerate 25 mg per day. Very few women are able to tolerate 50 mg. In cases of cancer, diabetes, severe adrenal deficiency, and autoimmune deficiency, I recommend that patients take the maximum dose they can tolerate. In the case of infertility, I recommend that women double their usual dose a few days before and after ovulation.

- **Increasing your DHEA supplement's efficacy.** First, always take DHEA with food. For better absorption, choose meals that comply with the principles of the ideal Natural Superwoman diet—lean protein, little or no grains and unfavorable carbohydrates, lots of vitamin-rich leafy green vegetables, and moderate amounts of fruits and healthy fats.

Apply the steps of the stress-release technology discussed in Chapter 11.

Supplement your diet with adaptogens, herbal supplements that balance the hormonal and immune system. An example of an herbal adaptogen is ginseng.

- **Possible side effects.** The earliest and most common side effect of DHEA treatment is agitation and a feeling of being hyper. You will be able to feel this side effect within the first to third day of beginning treatment or incrementally increasing your dose. If you begin treatment and immediately feel edgy, then you know you must reduce your dose. If you begin to feel agitated after the third day, but felt great in the first two days of initiating treatment or incrementally increasing your dose, you know that you should reduce your daily dose, but that you can use this higher dose when you anticipate having a more physically, emotionally, or mentally challenging day.

  The second most common side effect is oily skin and an acne-like breakout on your head, face, chest, neck, back, or buttocks. This oily skin and breakout may take one to three weeks to become apparent. For this reason I take great pains to recommend that women take their time and maintain their dose for at least two weeks before increasing it. If you find that you are breaking out, cease taking any DHEA, wait until your breakout passes, and then restart your treatment at the dose you tolerated before increasing and experiencing the breakout.

  More rare side effects are head hair loss and chin hair growth. These require one to three months to become apparent and most often occur among women who are generally prone to these side effects. For such women, I recommend they begin their treatment at the lowest dose and increase their dose even more slowly.

Finally, a less frequent side effect is the opposite-from-expected response, where women feel fatigued and depressed rather than the usual energetic and optimistic. This response is more likely in women who have very low levels of norepinephrine. In cases of opposite-from-expected response, DHEA treatment unexpectedly suppresses norepinephrine levels even further, causing these negative moods. In this situation, or in any other where taking DHEA produces unwanted results, immediately cut down or discontinue use and discuss your response with your health-care provider.

Remember, your body is as precious as a priceless Stradivarius violin. You cannot repair it with a sledgehammer. Be gentle and respond to its unique needs.

8 • Pregnenolone: Your Brain Power

QUICK QUIZ

Answer the following questions to find out if you may benefit from optimizing your pregnenolone levels:

Are you more forgetful lately?

Does your mind have trouble "rising" to a more challenging than usual mental task?

Are you not as sharp as you used to be, in general?

Do you no longer have the courage to share thoughts that are more controversial?

Is there a family history of Alzheimer's disease?

Do you have high cholesterol?

If so, do you use statin medications to treat and control it?

Do you take antianxiety medication and experience difficulty getting going in the morning?

Do you have difficulty seeing colors clearly?

Are you feeling more depressed than usual?

Do you have arthritis or do you experience joint pain?

Or, more generally, do you lack the vital physical energy you used to have?

If you identify with any of the conditions mentioned in these questions, you should consider exploring whether you are producing suboptimal levels of pregnenolone. Following are some of the reasons you may benefit from optimizing your levels.

PREGNENOLONE BASICS

In the 1950s, pregnenolone became fashionable as a miracle drug for treating rheumatoid arthritis. Extremely high doses—500 mg—were regularly prescribed to men and women alike. Soon after, the hormone cortisol was also discovered in the adrenal gland and proved to be a much more effective tool in treating arthritis. Pregnenolone treatment was abandoned and soon forgotten.

Historically, pregnenolone was regarded as the "mother of all hormones," as it was understood to participate in a chain of conversions that supplied our bodies with nearly all other hormones—progesterone, cortisol, DHEA, testosterone, and estrogen.

In my clinical experience with more than 3,000 patients supplementing pregnenolone, I have found that it is unusual—occasionally and rarely observed only in women under age eighteen—for supplementing pregnenolone to increase other hormone blood levels. In other words, I have found that actual blood testing and clinical response does not support the idea that pregnenolone is the source of all hormones. Instead, I have observed that pregnenolone is the key to your brain power. Pregnenolone directly improves your cognitive function in the following ways:

- **Makes you feel more alert** by suppressing GABA and increasing glutamate. At the same time, this amazing hormone protects you from the negative effects of increased glutamate by increasing dopamine and protecting your hippocampal brain cells from the amyloid beta protein, the dominant protein associated with Alzheimer's disease.

- **Increases your capacity for cognitive function** by developing and supporting your hippocampus, the thinking center of the brain.

- **Helps generate new brain cells.**

- **Actively supports overall memory** by increasing acetylcholine, the most dominant neurotransmitter associated with memory and cognitive function.

- **Increases spatial memory,** which provides you with the ability to physically navigate from one place to another.

- **Increases memory in the aged,** suggesting that it may reverse the effects of aging memory.

Do you think you don't need pregnenolone? Think again. While the most conservative data indicates that women lose 70 percent of their original production of pregnenolone by age sixty, my clinical experience indicates that this happens far earlier. I have observed that pregnenolone levels decline rapidly and early in life; it is not uncommon for me to see women in their twenties and thirties with no detectable levels of pregnenolone. Tests for measuring pregnenolone have responded to this dramatic drop. The two largest blood labs in the United States report that the normal range of pregnenolone for any age of life is 20 to 150 for one lab and 20 to 200 for the other. That's a dramatically broad range in my opinion. Amazingly, in my practice, the most common lab results I get—even for women in their twenties—is under twenty!

WHAT PREGNENOLONE CAN DO FOR YOU

By optimizing your pregnenolone levels, you will enjoy the following benefits:

- A reduction of cholesterol levels
- A boost in memory
- An increase in social confidence
- An occasional cognitive or intellectual boost
- A relief in hangovers and a next-day remedy when you've had too little sleep
- Less arthritis and joint pain

SUPPLEMENTING PREGNENOLONE TO ADDRESS SPECIFIC HEALTH ISSUES

Supplementing Pregnenolone to Increase Mental Focus and Memory

If you were to build a brain from scratch, you would start with pregnenolone. This hormone aids in the building, performance, and maintenance of your brain. Positive effects of pregnenolone include clear, sharp thinking.

As mentioned, in the 1950s, arthritis was treated with pregnenolone in high doses that would never be used today. These doses were taken by patients without reported side effects at the time of treatment. I mention this early use of pregnenolone only to underscore that the benefits of enhancing and maintaining memory function with pregnenolone come without side effects.

When supplementing pregnenolone to enhance memory, you must pay attention to your body. Any feeling of agitation or inability to focus means that you must reduce your dose.

Setting your dose. I generally ask patients to begin taking 50 mg with breakfast or lunch, and to increase both doses every two weeks. The maximum dosage I have recommended is 300 mg daily, although as I have said, historically arthritis patients have taken 500 mg daily. When you increase your dosage, watch how it affects you—you don't want to feel nervous or agitated. The moment you feel side effects, reduce your dosage. In order to do so most effectively, do not change your diet or intake of other supplements when you increase your dosage of pregnenolone; you want to know that any difference in the way you feel is related to your increase in pregnenolone.

Supplementing Pregnenolone to Increase Alertness and Social Confidence

- **Alertness.** One of the ways that antidepressant medications like Prozac and fluoxetine work is by increasing the level of pregnenolone in your brain. When you drink alcohol, the level of pregnenolone increases in your brain. This may not mean anything to you at first blush, but it evidences just how brilliant a woman's brain is. Alcohol acts as a sedative when consumed. As a result, your brain increases production of pregnenolone to decrease the sedative effect.

Your body also increases pregnenolone levels when you take medications like Valium (benzodiazepine), meant to relax and sedate you, to counteract the sedation, and help you stay more alert.

In other words, whatever sedation and alcohol take away from you, pregnenolone hands back to you.

This is incredible information. It seems that pregnenolone protects our brains from oversedation. It may be more useful than coffee on mornings when you wake up feeling drowsy. This morning, as I write this chapter with my daughter, I think about the fact that I went to bed late and began writing after only five hours of sleep. In addition to my coffee, I took 200 mg of pregnenolone.

I'm not advocating pregnenolone as a substitute for responsible alcohol consumption and a designated driver, nor do I endorse abusing pregnenolone supplements by regularly relying on pregnenolone to help you drive after an insufficient night's sleep. However, I do believe that once you know how, and at what doses, your body responds to pregnenolone, this natural hormone supplement can aid in increasing your level of alertness on an acute basis. In fact, I believe pregnenolone may be a great hangover remedy.

- **Social confidence.** People who have social phobias also have naturally low pregnenolone levels. In my own experience, pregnenolone injects a sense of cerebral chutzpah, or confidence. I have always felt a certain amount of shyness when accompanying my very social wife to parties populated by people I may not know. She seems to swim in the crowd, while I feel overwhelmed. When I began supplementing pregnenolone, I noticed that I began swimming too, and I was able to share myself in a way that had previously only been possible in small groups. Pregnenolone allowed me to express myself in larger groups without hesitation.

In general, pregnenolone reduces fear and increases social confidence in a unique way. For example, the hormone testosterone also decreases fear and increases confidence, but does so in an aggressive way. High levels of testosterone are associated with "bully" behavior and a sense of physical strength and superiority, even if the person feeling this way is not physically superior to an opponent. In my experience, pregnenolone decreases fear and increases social confidence in a manner that allows you to be the life of the party you had always known you could be.

Setting your dose. Unlike dosing instructions for other uses of pregnenolone, this hormone does not require you to take a steady dose to increase social confidence. Proper dosing of pregnenolone is individual. By beginning with the minimum recommended dose and seeing how your body reacts, in general, you can slowly increase the amount you take, and then tailor this dose to anticipate what you plan to do on a particular day or evening. For example, a morning dose may be perfect for days when you have a big meeting, but may agitate you on days you don't. The same dose may be ideal for a nighttime party, but may prevent you from falling asleep on a day when you plan a quiet evening at home. Begin with 50 mg per dose on a day when you do not have a social obligation and see what happens. Do you feel more outgoing and socially brave? Increase your dose until you do. Reduce your dosage the moment you feel agitated, nervous, or irritable. Once you have established how your body reacts to pregnenolone, supplement it when you require more cerebral chutzpah.

Supplementing Pregnenolone to Improve Eyesight

Pregnenolone is found in concentrated levels in the eye, especially in the retina, which it has also been shown to protect. Clinically, pregnenolone doesn't actually improve eyesight, but may increase your ability to see colors and details.

Setting your dose. You may follow general dosing guidelines to supplement pregnenolone for this purpose.

Supplementing Pregnenolone to Alleviate Joint Pain

Again, in the 1950s, 500 mg daily doses of pregnenolone were regularly prescribed to treat rheumatoid arthritis, with no side effects reported. My practice is not focused on rheumatoid arthritis patients and I do not prescribe pregnenolone in these quantities, but I personally find that I cannot take more than 300 mg without becoming edgy. Some of my patients reach that feeling at 50 mg. Even in the lower dose levels that I recommend for general pregnenolone supplementation, my patients have reported a decrease in joint pain.

Supplementing Pregnenolone to Reduce Cholesterol

Recent studies indicate that the presence of pregnenolone as part of an overall hormonal replacement program decreases total cholesterol levels. However, the statin medications currently prescribed to treat high cholesterol levels block your body's natural production of pregnenolone. The herbal alternative to statin, which is extracted from red Chinese rice, also partially blocks pregnenolone production. Clinically, it's rare to see a patient who takes statin medications and has any measurable level of pregnenolone, and there are many individual reports of memory loss associated with the use of statin medications. I have heard anecdotal patient reports of statin use causing alcohol consumption to affect them more strongly. Knowing how pregnenolone combats the sedative affects of alcohol consumption, this is not surprising.

Setting your dose. Practically, I recommend patients who take statin medications to consider supplementing pregnenolone at the maximum dose they can tolerate, not to exceed 300 mg daily.

Supplementing Pregnenolone to Improve Fertility

Pregnenolone plays an important role in the embryonic process, and I consider pregnenolone to be an important player in women's overall hormonal environment. So I incorporate pregnenolone in the treatment of patients wishing to increase fertility.

Setting your dose. Using pregnenolone in natural fertility-enhancement programs is highly individualized and requires the assistance of a health-care provider with experience in nutritional and hormonal protocols.

MORE DOSAGE INFORMATION

I recommend pregnenolone in the pill or sublingual drop form, but prefer the pill form, as it produces a longer-lasting effect in the body. The average patient under my care ultimately discovers that she benefits from 100 mg daily without side effects. I begin by recommending a dose of 50 mg at breakfast or lunch.

I encourage patients to increase their dose by 50 mg every two weeks and not change their diet or the dose of any other supplement in their individual program for one week of the initial or increased dose. This will allow you to be certain that the side effects you feel are related to your pregnenolone increase.

To enhance absorption, pregnenolone should be taken while consuming protein and healthy fats. As is the case when you supplement other hormones, taking pregnenolone on an empty stomach or with carbohydrates reduces the level of absorption.

- **Possible side effects**

Reduce your dosage if you feel hyper, irritable, agitated, or nervous. Side effects generally appear within a few hours or a few days of increasing your dose. In general, these side effects are mild, predictable, and possible to resolve as soon as you reduce your dosage. In some cases, you may experience a subtle decrease in your quality of sleep. Simply moving your midday dose to the morning or decreasing your dose will restore your previous sleep pattern.

On rare occasions, patients have reported experiencing slight shaking. This side effect is quickly resolved by ceasing all pregnenolone supplementation, waiting for the symptom to disappear, and restarting pregnenolone at a lower dose. Women with seizure-related conditions should be cautious when they supplement pregnenolone.

If you experience any unwanted side effects, I recommend reducing or omitting the dose.

 Rene's Story

Rene, forty, came to me and reported that for six months she had been taking statin medication to treat her high cholesterol. During this time she experienced some memory loss, and when asked, confirmed that alcohol began affecting her more strongly since she began her treatment course. In her blood tests, Rene's pregnenolone levels were undetectable, her cholesterol was low, but her triglycerides were still high. She did say that she consumes a high volume of high-glycemic carbohydrates.

I recommended that she replace her statin medication with Natural Superwoman eating, rich in low-glycemic carbohydrates, and pregnenolone supplements. She began taking 50 mg daily with breakfast and increased her dosage every two weeks. At 150 mg she began to feel agitated and decreased to a maintenance dose of 100 mg daily. Four months later, Rene returned to my office and confirmed that her memory "was back!" Her blood tests confirmed that her cholesterol had stayed within normal limits, despite the fact that she had stopped taking statin medication four months before. Additionally her HDL ("good" cholesterol) increased and her triglycerides decreased thanks to her new low-glycemic diet.

Chia's Story, Our Canine Family Member

Chia is our soon-to-be seventeen-year-old chow chow. Five years ago she began suffering from arthritis and slowed down substantially. The truth is, living to age twelve is a good life span for this large dog breed. Still, we felt that we could improve the quality of her remaining years by applying some of the hormonal technology my human patients enjoy. Consulting veterinary hormone studies, I learned that dogs are able to tolerate much higher levels of certain hormones. We began by giving her 25 mg of DHEA daily, with great response. Our friends laughed at us. Two years ago I increased her daily DHEA dose to 50 mg and then added 100 mg of pregnenolone daily and soon increased it to 200 mg daily. I noticed that she became increasingly more alert, social, and interested in her surroundings. In our household, we swear she tracks birds on television! Additionally, she began joining us for walks and then longer walks, which she had not done in years.

I share this story with you, not because I want to create a fashion of treating dogs with bioidentical hormones, but because it colors the discussion of pregnenolone efficacy. Chia has now far exceeded the life expectancy of the average chow chow and seems more youthful than she did five years ago prior to beginning her DHEA and pregnenolone treatment. She doesn't know about placebo effects, or about psychosomatic effects. She has simply responded favorably to a change to her hormonal profile.

9 • Testosterone: Your Secret Strength

When women hear the word "testosterone," they immediately want to know if supplementing testosterone will cause them to grow body hair. I explain that properly supplementing bioidentical testosterone does not cause women to develop male physical characteristics. Testosterone is a hormone that belongs to both men and women. It provides women with three important life tools:

- Empowers women with a feeling of confidence, security, and emotional strength.
- Restores women's athletic and physical function.
- Promotes a more proactive sense of sexuality.

Recently the FDA concluded that the concept of testosterone deficiency does not exist in women, and denied an application for the use of testosterone in the treatment of female sexual disorder. This conclusion was supported by a number of medical organizations.

This section discusses why the conclusion is incorrect from a scientific perspective, and why you have the right to define your sexual self and to choose other testosterone-related benefits by restoring your own level of bioidentical testosterone.

QUICK QUIZ

Many women are not aware of the symptoms of testosterone deficiency or testosterone overproduction. Answer the following questions to learn about both and how they may apply to you:

Quiz 1

Have you lost your sense of vitality? Love of life?

Do you experience feelings of insecurity?

Do you sometimes feel that you are not able to stand up to people? Did you used to be more assertive?

Do you have difficulty setting boundaries and saying no when others ask you to do things that stretch you too thin?

Do you find that you are less driven than you once were to engage in exercise? Does it seems that you always come up with an excuse to do something else?

Have you recently lost muscle mass? Gained weight?

Has your interest in sex declined?

Are your nipples and clitoris less sensitive than they used to be?

Does it take longer for you to reach orgasm?

Is your orgasm less intense than it used to be?

If you've had body hair in the past, do you notice that you have less of it now?

(continued)

Quiz 2

Have you noticed your hair thinning in the front and on top of your head, like a receding hairline?

Does your face feel more oily than usual?

Have you begun to get acne on your face or body, especially premenstrually and menstrually, if you still menstruate?

Have you been told you have adult acne?

Do your breakouts subside after you complete your period?

Do you feel agitated, especially premenstrually, and menstrually, impatient?

Do you surprise yourself by realizing that you're "looking" for conflict sometimes?

Do you find that you are less compromising than before? That you say no more than yes, in general?

If you find that you relate to the conditions described in Quiz 1, you are exhibiting the signs of testosterone deficiency. If you relate more to the conditions mentioned in Quiz 2, then your body is expressing the physical signs of excess testosterone. In the following sections you'll learn more about both of these testosterone profiles and, to the extent you choose to employ them, what's available to adjust the way you feel and function as a consequence.

TESTOSTERONE BASICS

Although we generally associate testosterone and other androgens with men, every woman produces testosterone, and every woman relies on testosterone to fulfill a myriad of hormonal and physiological functions. Obviously, some women naturally produce more testosterone, and therefore, are more athletic, have wider, flatter breasts, enjoy more muscle mass and definition, less body fat, more body hair, and have an assertive personality. Other women have lower testosterone profiles: they have higher-pitched voices, larger breasts, are less athletic, have minimal body hair, and have a more compromising disposition. Most women are a mix of the two.

UNDERSTANDING TESTOSTERONE EXPRESSION VERSUS BLOOD LEVELS

Uniquely, the expression of testosterone in women is not correlated to the level of testosterone measured in the bloodstream, as it is with men, but rather the amount of testosterone is found in target areas—in women's body tissue (paracrine) and within their cells (intracrine). How much does any woman have in these target areas? Unfortunately, a simple office blood test cannot establish the amount of cell and tissue testosterone that exists and so it cannot tell you whether treatment is necessary. However, you can use blood tests to monitor the course of an existing treatment. In the discussion to come, any time we talk about measuring testosterone by blood, we are referring to testosterone in the bloodstream and not the target areas mentioned above that determine testosterone's expression in women.

In men, most testosterone is circulated in the blood and acts globally. Conversely, most of the testosterone in a women's body is controlled and stored by a protein called sex-binding globulin, which holds or releases testosterone in reaction to estrogen levels. When estrogen levels decrease, sex-binding globulin releases more testosterone. Every woman reading this book who has, or once had, a regular menstrual cycle will be able to identify this process, as it is responsible for the hormonal "roller coaster" women experience every month.

This rise and fall of testosterone and estrogen levels is intimately related to your reproductive function. In the week after you finish your period, days six to thirteen of your cycle, estrogen levels rise and you experience the physical signs associated with balanced testosterone levels; your face clears up, and you feel and act softer and more compromising. During this week, your sexual feelings may be characterized as "romantic." On day fourteen, when you ovulate, your body sharply drops your estrogen levels, and within your target cells and tissue discussed above, your testosterone levels go sky-high, causing you to experience an aggressive need to be sexual. I call this "aggressive sexuality." It's a clarion call by your body. It is during there periods that you'll cancel your plans for a "girls' video night" in favor of a date or other opportunity to fertilize your waiting egg during the last hours of its availability.

A few days later, a week before your period returns, your estrogen levels begin to decline, as your body realizes that fertilization has not occurred, and, because of this drop, sex-binding globulin releases more stored testosterone for use in the target cells and tissue. During this week, you may feel more aggressive, impatient, more likely to raise your voice rather than compromise, and your skin may get oilier and break out in blemishes. You may also exhibit signs of estrogen decline, including insecurity, depression, and generally feeling blue. For more information on this process, see the section on estrogen and the hormone balance pillar (Chapter 4).

UNDERSTANDING TESTOSTERONE DEFICIENCY

Most of women's testosterone is produced in their ovaries. Women's testosterone expression peaks when they are in their early twenties and decreases by nearly 50 percent by the time they reach their mid-forties.

In January 2007, an alarming report in the main endocrine medical journal warned about a "substantial, yet unrecognized" recent decline in testosterone levels in men. To this clinician engaged in assisting both men and women in replenishing their falling testosterone supplies for many years, this was old news. In fact, however dramatic this phenomenon of falling testosterone levels is in men, it is only a fraction of what is happening to women. Women come to me every day, describing how their lives have been negatively affected by the symptoms that many of you may have related to in Quiz 1 (page 176). Nearly every day, I hear:

About self-confidence
"I've lost my sense of confidence."
"I don't know why I feel so insecure."

About physical activity and body image
"I always enjoyed it before, once I got into it, but now, somehow, I
    don't want to exercise, anymore."
"My upper arms feel droopy—I'm getting my grandmother's flabby
    arms!"

About sex drive
"I'd rather watch TV or sleep than have sex."
"I'm too old to focus on sex. I used to be so sexual, but now I never
    seem to be motivated."
"My partner and I still have sex, but I secretly hope he just finishes so
    I can get on with what I want to do."
"I'm dead sexually."
"It takes forever for me to reach orgasm these days, and then it's
    nothing compared to what it used to be."

I believe that the decline of testosterone's availability to women's bodies is significantly more dramatic than the decline in men's production. In the following pages, I'll explain how testosterone works and, if you choose, how and why you may naturally supplement your current available testosterone.

HOW TESTOSTERONE BENEFITS WOMEN

If you've never considered testosterone to be an important hormone in your life as a woman, or if you've feared that testosterone would compromise your health or femininity, this section will be particularly interesting to you. Testosterone provides women with health and quality of life benefits across the four pillars.

The top three reasons to be enthusiastic about testosterone are improved sexual arousal and response; emotional confidence; and natural athletic performance.

- **Testosterone restores and improves your sexual arousal and response.** When testosterone is given to women immediately following removal of their ovaries (as we discussed, when women's ovaries are removed, women lose 70 percent of their testosterone nearly overnight), if applied topically, these women do not lose their sexual function—their hormonal and testosterone health does not skip a beat. Absent this, restoration of sexual function and response is a major issue in the lives and full recovery of this group. By simply applying testosterone, along with estrogen, topically immediately after surgery, the issue of sexual interruption and dysfunction becomes a nonissue. Testosterone has also been shown to benefit the sexuality of women who have not undergone hysterectomy or removal of their ovaries. The effect is physical, not simply psychological. The amount of testosterone supplemented directly correlates to the growth or shrinkage of a specific area of the brain.

I have treated more than 4,000 women with testosterone over the last twenty years. Close to a thousand of my current patients use testosterone. On the basis of their responses, I believe that testosterone treatment should be made available to women, irrespective of whether they have undergone hysterectomy, have had their ovaries removed, or are in menopause or perimenopause. Testosterone should be given to any woman who is searching for a remedy to a decrease in her sexual function and response. There is only one contraindication, or situation where testosterone should not be administered, and that situation is a clinical sign of excess testosterone.

If you have hair on your chin, oily skin, acne, receding hairline, and if you are prone to physically aggressive tendencies, you may not be a candidate for supplementing testosterone. Women in this group already have enough testosterone in their target areas, and in my experience, their sex drive will improve (in addition, their acne, oily skin, chin hair, receding hairline, and physical aggression will resolve) when they are treated with estrogen.

If you believe that you need assistance in restoring your sexual function and response, the guidelines outlined in the sections that follow will instruct you on how to safely supplement testosterone. If you do experience any side effects, these will be limited to those listed above, and all are immediately controllable if you simply curb your dose.

- **Testosterone helps you live with a feeling of well-being and confidence.** Testosterone gives women an overall feeling of safety and security, by helping them manage fear. In studies, one dose of testosterone significantly reduced women's physiological fear response. In my experience, women who complain of feeling too timid, submissive, or insecure greatly benefit from treatment with testosterone. In fact, women who familiarize themselves with ideal doses on an individual basis are able to use testosterone situationally, say, before a big workday when they need extra courage, before a big party when they know they must force themselves to mingle, or before an important professional or personal confrontation when they must be clearheaded and strong in order to properly express their thoughts and feelings.

- **Testosterone builds your muscle tone and increases your athletic ability.** As it does in men, testosterone plays a role in muscle development. In women who have experienced muscular decline, restoring testosterone levels also restores their muscle tone and ability to perform athletically. In my experience, testosterone restores the declining physical function that comes with age—promoting overall strength, increasing muscle strength, decreasing muscle fatigue following workout, and improving hand-eye coordination and balance.

Testosterone should never be used to "overbuild" muscle development beyond natural predisposition. I believe the misuse of testosterone by men is destructive, but in women, misuse is destructive physiologically and also catastrophic to their physical and psychological feminine identity. Women misusing testosterone can lose their breast tissue, grow hair in all the wrong places (face, chest, back, arms), and lose hair on their heads.

When used responsibly, women's use of testosterone will not cause them to build muscle size the way it does in men. Physiological replacement of testosterone in women simply restores what has been lost, meaning you had to have had it once in order for testosterone to rebuild it.

MORE BENEFITS OF TESTOSTERONE

In addition to the three major, immediate benefits, testosterone also supports the body in numerous ways. Testosterone:

- **Helps battle depression.** Studies indicate that for many women, simply restoring their sexual function with testosterone alleviates some measure of depression. In addition, there is compelling data that testosterone supplementation itself has a positive effect on depression. I frequently see women on selective serotonin reuptake inhibitor (SSRI) medications who complain that they have lost their sexual desire and response as a result of taking these antidepressant medications. Testosterone is able to help these women's conditions, but their response is not as strong as women who do not take SSRI. When estrogen is added to this testosterone treatment, both the depression and sexual response improve significantly. In the cases of clinically depressed men treated with SSRI medications, the addition of testosterone to this treatment protocol significantly improves their depression and sexual function.

In my experience, testosterone is a tremendous antidepressant tool, generally promoting a feeling of confidence and well-being, sexual function and response, and improved athletic ability. Simply promoting these feelings goes a long way toward uplifting a depressed person's outlook.

- **Alleviates "cluster" headaches.** Treatment with testosterone, combined with estrogen and melatonin, has been shown to have a significantly beneficial effect on this hard-to-treat headache.

- **Protects bone health.** Testosterone is known to be a great bone builder in both men and women. In general, women with bone loss due to osteoporosis do not break their bones unless they fall. Testosterone is the substance they require to avoid both the fall and the fracture. Testosterone improves balance, making it less likely that women will fall, and also promotes hand-eye coordination, so women are able to brace themselves in order to avoid or minimize injury if they do fall. Additionally, testosterone bolsters muscle development around the bone—effectively creating a cushion that protects the bone during a fall. And finally, testosterone actually builds new bone. While estrogen and most medications may help prevent bone loss, only testosterone and human growth hormone actually build bone.

I commonly help women improve their bone density by adding testosterone to their natural hormonal treatment program.

- **Promotes fertility.** Women undergoing in vitro fertilization (IVF) who have not responded to treatment enjoy improved results when testosterone is added to their program. I recommend supplementing testosterone because it supports follicle development, an essential component of the successful conception process. A physician with experience in treating infertility with bioidentical hormones can instruct you on the specific, highly individualized supplement method and time of the cycle for the treatment of infertility with testosterone.

ADDRESSING CONCERNS ABOUT TESTOSTERONE

Many women would like to maximize these aspects of their lives, but are concerned with reports about using testosterone putting them at risk of certain diseases or becoming more masculine. When women supplement testosterone properly, as is outlined in the section on setting the dose, they do not develop masculine characteristics. You will learn more about this in the section on supplementing testosterone at the end of this chapter (page 191). The following section directly addresses why testosterone does not put you at risk of developing other health concerns.

- **Testosterone and cardiovascular disease.** Testosterone does not exacerbate cardiovascular disease, and may even provide protective benefits to the cardiovascular system. In men, testosterone treatment provides measurable cardiovascular benefits. In women, testosterone provides similar, but less significant assistance. When women age and enter menopause, the associated decrease in testosterone levels results in decreased blood flow in the arteries and an increased thickness of the carotid artery walls. In studies on mice treated with testosterone, coronary artery function improved. In many studies, researchers follow female-to-male transsexual patients who receive years of testosterone supplements ten- to fifteenfold higher than their naturally occurring testosterone. In fact, this is one of the most closely monitored groups in the world of hormone treatment. Research has not shown a rise in heart disease. In other words, testosterone neither harms nor provides significant benefit to a woman's cardiovascular health, and therefore should not be a source of concern for your supplement program.

- **Testosterone and diabetes.** Testosterone does not cause diabetes. In men, testosterone treatment is extremely helpful in preventing and treating diabetes. However, in women, there is a general concern regarding supplementing testosterone and diabetes due to information about women with polycystic ovaries. Women in this group can be hairy, have highly developed musculature, and have relatively higher levels of testosterone. They also have a tendency toward obesity and diabetes. There is a fear that the relatively high incidence of diabetes in these women is related to testosterone. However, research shows that these women have unique defects that cause their polycystic syndrome, and that simply losing weight reverses their prediabetic tendencies. In female-to-male transsexual patients, years of very large doses of testosterone relative to natural female levels have no affect on insulin sensitivity.

  In my experience treating women with testosterone and closely monitoring their sugar, insulin, and hemoglobin A1c levels, I have never observed any changes in improvement or deterioration of the prediabetic condition.

- **Testosterone and breast cancer.** Testosterone does not cause, and in fact *protects,* against breast cancer. Any woman who discusses testosterone therapy with me always begins the conversation by asking me whether supplementing testosterone will make her look like a man, and whether supplementing testosterone will cause breast cancer.

  Breast cancer is the number one hot-button issue whenever anyone speaks about supplementing any hormone. Testosterone treatment does not cause or aggravate breast cancer; it is also a strong tool for preventing and protecting against breast cancer. To date, there has not been a single case reported wherein a female-to-male transsexual who received testosterone treatment developed breast cancer. Scientific literature is rich with information on the protective effects of androgens, including testosterone, on breast cancer.

In my clinic, I have not observed any link between testosterone supplementation and breast cancer. In fact, women with breast cancer can safely supplement testosterone to alleviate other symptoms.

WHY THE CONTROVERSY OVER TESTOSTERONE?

Despite the fact that testosterone has been proven to be safe, officially the FDA does not recognize its benefits.

Women's sex drive is at the core of today's testosterone controversy. Significant numbers of women report diminished sex drives. In fact, even if blood levels were indicative of the amount of testosterone available, medicine's ability to measure testosterone blood levels is known to be inaccurate—results are often falsely high due to common manufacturing errors in calibration. Yet the FDA and the larger medical establishment will not accept this as a reason to approve testosterone supplementation in women, as diminished sex drive does not always correlate with diminished testosterone *blood levels*. As discussed, the amount of testosterone available to women—their testosterone *expression*—does not correlate with the amount of testosterone in their blood but rather the amount found in their cell tissue.

Are women misrepresenting their sexual response in order to "dope" on testosterone? Are they sex addicts looking for recreational sex aids? Hardly. The medical community's inability to properly measure testosterone in women misclassifies them. And, of course, there is also the matter of women's testosterone levels naturally falling between ages twenty and forty.

By denying approval of a process to treat women's sexual dysfunction with testosterone, claiming that, as a general group, women are not testosterone deficient and require no mechanism to enhance their levels of testosterone, the FDA failed to recognize the unique way in which testosterone expresses itself in women. Let's take a look at the other ways the studies used by the FDA were flawed.

- **FDA review did not take into account women who take birth control pills.** When women take oral contraceptives (birth control pills), the presence of the chemicalized hormones in the pill causes the ovaries to stop making estrogen and progesterone, in favor of the chemicalized medication delivered every day. This also affects the production level of other hormones produced by the ovaries, and the net effect is that testosterone levels are reduced by 70 percent. This effect is seen at any age. In addition, oral contraceptives significantly increase the level of sex-binding globulin, resulting in a further decline of available testosterone expression.

The effect that oral contraceptives have on testosterone levels is devastating. In my own practice I have observed that, irrespective of their "peak" sexual age, women who stop taking birth control pills are not able to resurrect the testosterone levels they enjoyed prior to starting the pill. My strong feeling is that oral contraceptives have a lasting effect on the ovaries' ability to produce testosterone in general.

Two new "developments" in the world of the birth control pill do not address, and may further exacerbate, this concern.

In the first development that is intended to address the side effects associated with the placebo week of the pill, women are advised to skip the placebo week and begin immediately taking the new month's supply, so that they are constantly taking "active" pills. This exacerbates the phenomenon discussed above.

In the second development, women who experience the significant hormonal decreases associated with perimenopause are instructed to take birth control pills because they are "better for them," rather than being advised to boost their declining levels with bioidentical hormones. For these women, between the testosterone decline that caused them to seek advice in the first place and, now, the 70 percent decline associated with taking the birth control pill, the effective testosterone expression available to them is very nearly zero.

Between these two recommendations and the phenomenon described in the estrogen section, where young girls are advised to control premenstrual symptoms by taking the birth control pill even if they are not sexually active, we have somehow entered an era where women are encouraged to take birth control pills forever. And in doing so, they also forfeit their natural production and benefits of testosterone.

- **FDA review also did not take into account women who have had their ovaries removed.** Many women over age forty are advised to remove their ovaries during hysterectomy in order to prevent ovarian cancer. What these women are *not* told is that, as a group, the women who elect to do so have a *higher* incidence of cardiovascular disease and a decline in cognitive function. Within seventy-two hours of the time their ovaries are removed, women in this group lose 70 percent of their testosterone level. In my experience, women who have had their ovaries removed in this way, and who are not put on bioidentical hormones immediately after their surgery, experience an alarmingly severe response to the near-instant and abrupt change in their hormone levels. Because of this hormone lapse and associated trauma, I find that this group can be the most difficult to assist in regaining their hormonal balance. If you must consider this type of prophylactic surgery, make sure to have your estrogen, progesterone, and testosterone levels checked prior to your procedure and then insist on receiving bioidentical replacement for these levels in *the day after* your surgery—not a week, a month, or a year after. In my experience, hours can make a difference in your ability to regain your hormonal health.

- **FDA review did not take into account studies with non-bioidentical hormones.** Most of the studies on supplementing estrogen and testosterone were conducted using Premarin, not bioidentical estrogen. As discussed in Chapter 4, Premarin is known to increase your level of sex-binding globulin. By doing so, Premarin decreases the amount of testosterone available to you, thereby making it impossible for you to enjoy any of the benefits of supplementing testosterone, and also making it impossible for the authors of the study to demonstrate that women enjoy benefits by adding testosterone to their hormonal profiles.

- **FDA review did not take into account studies on users of antidepressants.** Many of you have been offered Prozac for any one of a dozen conditions at some point in your life. Some women who elect to begin taking Prozac and other medications like Zoloft, and others in the SSRI family do improve significantly. Other women simply feel numb. A good percentage find that they don't respond at all. Irrespective of whether Prozac helps women, an absolute majority in all three groups lose some portion of their sexual drive and function as a consequence of taking this medication. In my experience, women on SSRI medications who are given testosterone to address their sexual side effects do not respond as well. In the case of these women, their dampened sexual response is not due to lowered testosterone levels. So, obviously, in studies that test whether testosterone treatment can assist women who have lost their sexual function due to SSRI treatment, testosterone will not present well.

CHEMICALIZED TESTOSTERONE

The only FDA-approved testosterone is a chemicalized form of testosterone called methyltestosterone. This medication is not identical to the testosterone produced by your body. It is also toxic to your liver and has been banned in a number of countries. Measurements taken during treatment with this drug are not relevant to treatments that use natural testosterone. And yet, this and the foregoing is the science used by the FDA to assess testosterone treatment. How can this be the standard used by the governmental agency charged with informing Americans about safe treatment options?

These faulty studies have caused the medical establishment to conclude that it is not possible to settle on a precise definition of androgen deficiency in women on the basis of blood tests, and that there is no established "normal range" for testosterone and other androgens in women.

In essence, they've concluded that it is not possible to make an educated assessment about the very existence of an androgen (testosterone and DHEA) deficiency in women. The reality is that women are not making this stuff up—and that second-guessing them about whether they are androgen deficient, and therefore whether compromised sexual response actually exists, is patronizing and insulting to women everywhere.

SUPPLEMENTING TESTOSTERONE

- **Available forms and efficacy.** Bioidentical testosterone is available in an injectable form, sublingual (under the tongue), in pill form, and in transdermal creams or gels and patches. In the United States, the testosterone patch is not available to women because, as explained in the previous sections, the FDA and various medical associations that recommend hormone uses contend that women cannot benefit from supplementing this hormone.

I do not recommend the bioidentical testosterone found in pill form, as it decreases women's level of HDL, the "good" cholesterol, and fails to yield results that are as good as other forms. I also do not recommend methyltestosterone, a chemicalized testosterone approved by the FDA for use by women and available in pill form, because it has been found to be toxic to the liver.

In my practice, I limit use to bioidentical testosterone in cream or gel and sublingual forms. I do not use injectables because the effect of this delivery mechanism lasts for weeks and months, making it more difficult to tweak your dose in the event you have used too much. By contrast, the sublingual form reaches peak effect within fifteen minutes of use and restores preapplication levels within two hours. When applied vaginally, studies indicate that cream or gel testosterone peaks at five and a half hours and lasts for more than twelve hours. These reports are consistent with efficacy times reported for general skin application, rather than specifically for vaginal application. When women apply testosterone cream or gel vaginally, specifically to the areas that I recommend, the clinical peak—in time and effect—is much greater. Beyond this, the mental and physical response lasts for many more hours because, as I've explained, testosterone expression is likely determined by what happens when testosterone enters our cells, rather than the level of testosterone in our blood.

- **How and when to supplement.** Every inch of your skin, besides the palms of your hands, the soles of your feet, and your small labia, will grow hair if testosterone is applied to it. For this reason, I suggest that women apply testosterone cream or gel directly onto the soles of their feet, after they shower in the morning or at night when feet are able to absorb the cream or gel. The cream or gel I recommend has a great absorption rate and provides patients with desired results.

To further enhance sexual response, I also recommend women apply testosterone cream or gel directly onto the small labia, clitoris, and G-spot before sexual activity. In application studies, women continued to report genital arousal three to four hours after peak effect.

- **For prolapse of the rectum and bladder.** In the majority of hysterectomies performed in the United States, the uterus and also the cervix are removed. The result is that the roof of the vagina is absent, leading to more common prolapse of the rectum and bladder into the vagina. For these women, I recommend a daily application of testosterone cream or gel internally, to the general area just under the bladder, found approximately one or two inches inside the vagina, along the top. In my experience, applying testosterone in this way helps to strengthen the musculature of the pelvis, vagina, and bladder neck, and prevent prolapse. I also suggest topical application to manage and decrease the consequences of prolapse when it occurs. Finally, I recommend topical vaginal application in the case of stress incontinence and have found it to be helpful to women with this condition.

- **Setting your dose.** Ideal doses vary individually based on how efficiently your body responds to the cream or gel or sublingual drop forms. In my practice, the cream or gel I use is 0.6 percent per gram (providing 6 mg per gram), the sublingual drops 0.5 mg per one drop. The average woman reaches her optimal result with half a gram of cream or gel once or twice per day. A minority of women require a gram and a half once or twice a day.

  With sublingual drops, the average women requires four drops under the tongue, once or twice a day, and a minority of women require up to ten drops, once or twice a day.

  When beginning your testosterone treatment, begin with the lowest dose—one-eighth or one-quarter gram of the cream or gel or one or two drops, once or twice a day. Your incremental increases should be slow, every two to three weeks, and should not exceed one-eighth or one-quarter of a gram of cream or gel, or one to two drops, once or twice a day. Stop increasing your dose when you experience side effects or if you reach your desired goal. Do not exceed one gram or ten drops, once or twice a day.

POSSIBLE SIDE EFFECTS

Upon learning the side effects of testosterone, most women immediately think of the East German Olympic Team of the past—women whose bodies had lost their feminine appearance. I want to reassure every woman reading this book, that if you use testosterone in the manner specified here, any side effects you experience will be mild, recognized, and arrested early. Side effects associated with testosterone include:

- **Aggressive behavior.** This includes feeling more aggressive or impatient than usual, or finding that you are shouting more often. This side effect presents itself within a few hours of taking a dose that is a bit too high for you. To manage this side effect, simply decrease your dose.

An important note on being "aggressive": If throughout your life you have been less assertive than others, and often did not have the confidence to express how you feel, or have agreed with others when you preferred to disagree, determining what "aggressive behavior" is for you requires additional consideration. Often, compliant people tend to keep company with people who benefit from the fact that they are willing to bend, even when they'd rather not. In other words, some people take advantage. Before lowering your dose of testosterone because someone has told you that you are being "too assertive" or even "bitchy," consult with the person in your life who is always encouraging you to be more brave and to stand up for yourself. Don't let bullies rob you of your newfound voice simply because it is convenient for them.

On the other hand, there are days when your schedule demands more testosterone of you than usual; for example, a tennis game, a relatively easy hike that you previously had problems completing, or a day when you must brace yourself for a conflict. Once you establish your ideal daily dose, you will be able to slightly increase your dose for more challenging days, on a day-to-day and case-by-case basis.

- **Oily skin and acne-like breakouts.** Testosterone-related oiliness and breakouts usually appear on the face, but on some women may appear only on buttocks, back, chest, neck, or head. This side effect generally takes two to three weeks to appear. In women who are prone to oily skin and acne-like breakouts, it may appear in only one week. To remedy this, stop using your testosterone supplement altogether. You may resume using testosterone once you observe that your oily skin and breakouts resolve. Begin by using a dose that is 25 percent lower than the one you used before you experienced this side effect, or use the same dose once, versus twice a day, or use the same dose, but skip days.

An important note about breakouts: Women whose breakouts are on their buttocks or on the top of their heads but who otherwise really enjoy the benefits associated with their dose may be inclined to continue using this dose, in spite of the out-of-view side effect. *This is a mistake.* Women should not ignore their bodies' expression of *any* unwanted side effects, which are your body's way of telling you that you have exceeded your personal ideal dose. In the longer term, women who ignore these side effects risk losing hair on their heads and begin growing hair on their chins and other body parts.

One way to avoid breakouts and continue using a dose that provides you with the feeling of confidence you desire is to use this dose once, versus twice a day, or to alternate days.

- **Body hair.** Whenever you apply testosterone cream or gel to an area of the body, other than the areas I specified, you may grow hair in that area, and *only* in that area.

- **Head hair loss and facial hair growth.** As indicated above, if you persist in using a dose that is higher than what your body prefers, and ignore the side effects of oily skin and breakouts, you may begin to lose hair on your head and grow hair on your chin and then on other parts of your body where you currently have hair. To remedy this, *stop using your testosterone supplement altogether.* You may resume using testosterone once you observe that you no longer lose head hair. Begin by using a dose that is 25 percent lower than the one you used when you began losing hair. If you have grown hairs on your chin, try applying estrogen gel to the affected area. Recent studies report that caffeine may also be helpful in counteracting head hair loss.

An important note on women's hair loss unrelated to supplementing testosterone: The general issue of hair loss in women is problematic and difficult to resolve. While it is beyond the scope of this book, I caution that medications like Propecia, designed to control hair loss by preventing testosterone from converting to DHT, present a larger hormonal problem. These medications also prevent progesterone from converting into allopregnenolone, an essential physiological conversion. A growing body of data raises significant concern that these medications may cause neurodegenerative disease. For this reason, I caution women to think twice before turning to systemic medications like Propecia to remedy their hair loss.

- **Unusual side effects from overuse.** I recommend that women limit their daily testosterone dose to a maximum of one gram twice a day. Studies indicate that *significantly* exceeding this recommended dose for supplementing testosterone can lower the tone of your voice and increase the size of your clitoris. Using the application techniques outlined above, I have never observed a woman under my care experiencing these conditions. Women with these side effects who were referred to my practice by others are able to resolve these conditions within a few short months by significantly decreasing their doses.

On the other hand, the section on estrogen discusses how an estrogen level decrease causes an increase of testosterone in the cells. One of my relatively young patients who works as a professional mezzo-soprano in an opera company complained that she began to lose her high soprano voice. Supplementing bioidentical estrogen restored her high-pitched voice.

I strongly condemn the use of testosterone to develop muscle growth beyond a woman's natural physiological scope.

Testosterone is a major player in your body's hormonal system. As with most hormones, your body's natural level of production and the benefits you enjoy may decline with the passage of time. It is your right and your choice to retain and regain the advantages that you have lost.

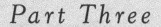

Part Three

Natural Superwoman Strategies for Balancing Mood

10 • The Power of Neurotransmitters

MIND AND MOOD MANAGEMENT FOR THE NATURAL SUPERWOMAN

We all want to feel great as often as possible, but do you know anyone who enjoys constant good moods, every day? The very notion contradicts the fact that human beings come equipped with a full emotional range. Why else would our bodies and minds have developed such a complex interactive system to address our various moods? Instead, the majority of us may be generally organized into three "mood profiles":

- **The mood disorder group.** Women in this group share a frustration that their lives seem to be controlled by constant, sometimes daily, mood disorders, including depression, anxiety, restlessness, and insomnia.

- **The mood cycle group.** This group experiences fairly consistent, periodic negative moods. And while these negative moods do not *control* their lives, they are annoying enough to make these women feel less productive than they'd like to be.

- **The occasional mood group.** Finally, others of us experience intermittent and mild mood disturbances. Many people have theories about why we're plagued by stress, occasional insomnia, and other maladies; my theory is simply that it is difficult to live in a fast-paced high-tech world while inhabiting a body designed for low-tech conditions. As sophisticated as our bodies are, they're still old technology.

Whatever your personal mood profile, you will find tools for identifying and addressing negative moods. The tools described in this chapter:

- Include natural remedies or applications.
- Have no drug-related side effects when properly administered.
- Will allow you to predict how you will feel and, for the most part, allow you to control your own dosage based on your schedule and personal rhythm.

All of this is so you can make your life more like the way you want it to be, every day. That's what it means to be a Natural Superwoman. It's not that a Natural Superwoman doesn't have bumps in the road, it's that she has natural tools at her disposal to make her life function at its personal best, despite those bumps.

NATURAL HEALING FOR MOOD?

Our body comes equipped with wonderful natural tools. With them, a woman's body is able to overcome the most difficult challenges known to humankind: starvation, environmental stress (i.e., inadequate temperature control), and natural predators (animals competing for food). If our equipment is meant to function under these torturous conditions, it stands to reason that we can adapt it to our everyday needs when circumstances are not so dire. In other words, however jam-packed the day that lies ahead of you—juggling work, kids, friends, your partner—recognize that without consulting a single time-management book, you already have all you need within you to manage your day, your week, and your life. *You* have the ability to make yourself feel that you are in control of your world. This natural coding is true for every woman reading this book. By contrast, *no* woman reading this book was born with a natural deficiency of Prozac, Xanax, or Ambien. So why not give your own body's remedy the first shot?

WHY ARE "NATURAL" TOOLS IN NEED OF TWEAKING?

If it's true that your body is fully equipped to handle nearly anything, why do you feel like you do? Many women suffer from negative moods because their systems are not functioning optimally due to poor diet, exposure to environmental toxins, emotional, physical, or professional stress, insufficient or excessive physical activity, declining natural hormones, or overmedication. Whatever your reasons, by simply incorporating a few key *four pillar* principles, you can regain control of your mind and mood in a meaningful way. First, let's understand how mood works biologically.

WHAT IS MOOD, ANYWAY?

Mood is many things, but on a scientific basis, mood is a reaction to a dance by neurotransmitters, those chemicals that deliver messages from one brain cell to another. This is the biochemical essence of all of our thoughts, emotions, and reactions. To understand how they work, we must first understand what primary neurotransmitters control mood, and what we can do to promote the increase, decrease, or balance of their levels—allowing us to control how often we feel good, naturally.

For the purposes of this discussion, I will focus on six neurotransmitters—two amino acids (glutamate and GABA) and four monoamines (dopamine, serotonin, norepinephrine, and epinephrine)—and explain what components of the *four pillars* affect each of these.

GETTING TO KNOW MOOD-RELATED NEUROTRANSMITTERS AND HOW THE FOUR PILLARS AFFECT THEM

The following description of primary neurotransmitters includes information on ideal diet and supplements that affect the levels of each. A more thorough discussion of how you can use the principles of all four pillars to remedy a variety of conditions follows in the later parts of this section. Some neurotransmitters you want to increase:

- **GABA (gamma-aminobutyric acid)** is an "inhibitor," a calming neurotransmitter that also controls motor behavior. Low levels of GABA are associated with anxiety and excessive worrying, depression, insomnia, and restlessness.

- **Serotonin.** This inhibitory, or calming, neurotransmitter begins as L-tryptophan—the amino acid found in milk and turkey known for encouraging sleep—and converts into 5-hydroxytryptophan (5-HT) in order to cross the brain barrier, where it becomes serotonin. Once in the brain, serotonin produces a calming mood and also converts to melatonin, which helps you to fall asleep and enjoy better-quality sleep. Low serotonin levels are associated with depression, insomnia, obsessive-compulsive disorder (OCD), anxiety, migraine, substance abuse, poor diet, increased appetite, craving for sweets, and increased inflammation. Increasing serotonin nutritionally helps significantly reduce depression and anxiety.

- **Dopamine.** Dopamine is a stimulating, nonagitating neurotransmitter charged with increasing our focus, attention, learning memory, sexual behavior, and fine motor movements. At optimum levels, dopamine improves motivation and acts as a strong antioxidant, curbing the destruction of brain cells. On the other hand, when your dopamine levels are low, you are likely to experience fatigue, low motivation, depression, decreased sex drive, increased incidents of substance abuse, Parkinson's disease, attention deficit disorders (ADD/ADHD), and restless leg syndrome.

- **Glutamate.** Glutamate is a major excitatory (noncalming) neurotransmitter. It plays an important role in our brain's ability to adapt to our environment, controls our ability to learn, and is essential for making new brain connections. On the other hand, elevated levels of glutamate decrease the flow of oxygen to our brains, causing neuron destruction. Too much glutamate very literally *kills* brain cells. High glutamate is associated with neurodegenerative diseases and conditions, including migraine, seizures, Lou Gehrig's disease, Parkinson's, and Alzheimer's.

Sounds bad, right? It is, but don't allow yourself to become stressed in thinking about this, because simply experiencing stress and physical trauma significantly increases levels of glutamate.

Instead, take a deep breath. Complete, regulated breathing—and a general increase in taking in oxygen—is essential for combating the destructive consequences associated with experiencing stress. You'll learn more about how breathing can lower glutamate levels in the section on breathing in Chapter 11.

Beyond breathing, our brain has a great system for moderating glutamate levels—like our immune system that sends out white blood cells to fight disease and infection, our brain sends out astrocytes to trap and destroy excess glutamate.

- **Norepinephrine and epinephrine.** Both norepinephrine and epinephrine are excitatory, or stimulating, neurotransmitters synthesized in the adrenal gland by the conversion of dopamine and another enzyme. Most of us have ten times more norepinephrine than epinephrine.

  Norepinephrine helps us maintain focus and attention and increases when we experience stress. Epinephrine stimulates perspiration, a rise in blood sugar, constriction of arteries, rising blood pressure, heart rate, and blood flow to essential organs, brain, heart, and muscles. Epinephrine increases with stress, fear, anger, fight-or-flight responses, and other physical trauma.

  When we experience constant stress, we also chronically increase epinephrine and begin developing related chronic high blood pressure, insulin deficiency, stress, and insomnia. On the other hand, when norepinephrine and epinephrine dip to levels that are too low, we experience fibromyalgia, pain, anorexia, bulimia, and depression. For this reason, epinephrine levels must be balanced—not too high, not too low.

  The psychopharmacological treatment of depression and anxiety is often a hit-or-miss process that requires your mental health professional to prescribe a number of medications that are known to increase serotonin, dopamine, and other neurotransmitters, and then see how you feel. Each of these medications has various sexual and other side effects.

  The reason this process seems so imprecise is because *it is*. Science has not yet identified a means of precisely measuring neurotransmitter levels. In other words, your doctor is somewhat in the dark—he or she doesn't have an exact baseline of neurotransmitter levels from which to start, so he or she begins with the basics, sees how you feel, and adds or subtracts from there.

New technology is currently being developed in an attempt to use urine testing to measure neurotransmitter levels.

In my practice, I use the whole range of natural supplements listed in this chapter to increase, decrease, or balance the neurotransmitter I believe each patient requires. The process is highly individualized and requires the participation and daily (sometimes hourly) monitoring by the patient herself. When used properly, these natural supplements may be effective and do not produce side effects. My preference is to try these natural remedies first and encourage you to consider doing the same.

A more thorough discussion of how the ideal diet and nutritional supplement, hormone, mind and mood, and activity maintenance pillars assist in remedying specific mind and mood conditions follows in the discussion of each condition.

APPLYING THESE NATURAL REMEDIES TO SPECIFIC MIND AND MOOD CONDITIONS

Once you understand how four-pillar technology—the nutrients you consume, what hormones your body is operating with, how you feel, and what activities you engage in—affects your brain chemistry, you can directly apply these natural remedies to address specific mind and mood conditions that control, slow down, or simply annoy you from time to time. The chapters that follow specifically address how you can apply this information to minimize stress, depression, anxiety, insomnia, and lapses in your memory.

11 • Relieving Stress

QUICK QUIZ

Answer the following questions to find out if you may benefit from reducing your stress level:

Do you find that you must catch your breath often?

Does your mind race?

Do you have memory lapses? Do small details slip your mind? Or is your memory cloudy?

Do you feel tense and anxious during relaxing times?

Do you become impatient or agitated over things that wouldn't have been such a big deal in the past?

Do you feel relaxed by physical activity, or does it exhaust you?

Are you exhausted by emotional interactions?

Do you have difficulty falling asleep?

Do you wake up feeling wired, your mind racing, and earlier than you'd like to?

Do you find yourself craving or eating more sweets, carbohydrates, or spicy or salty foods than usual?

Do you find it hard to sit still?

Do you eat quickly? Does it seem that you swallow your food too quickly to taste it?

Are you fidgety?

Have you been drinking more caffeine, sodas, or alcohol lately?

Are you experiencing more conflicts in your relationships than usual?

Are you sensitive to loud noise? Do you find that you cannot tolerate noise, even for a short period of time?

Do you have a hard time transitioning to environmental changes, such as cold to hot, dry to humid?

Do you feel generally negative? More emotional outbursts than usual? More dramatic than is usual?

If you used to like to travel, do you find that your ability to plan and execute even short "adventures" is limited?

Are you experiencing more hair loss than usual?

Have you found more brown spots on your face recently?

If you pull down your lower eyelid, is the flesh more red than usual?

Is your body temperature higher than usual?

Do your hands and feet perspire more than usual, even without physical activity?

If many of these conditions match your recent experience, your level of stress has begun to affect your health and performance, and must be brought under control.

Uzzi's Stress Journey

Some of us eat too much, a few of us eat too little; some exercise too much, others not enough; some are too stressed, others are so relaxed that they are withdrawn; some cannot sleep, others sleep too much; some don't integrate sexuality into their lives, others prioritize sexuality to the detriment of other pastimes; some of us focus on work to the exclusion of hobbies, and others are so focused on leisure activities that we are not able to do our work properly.

In other words, few of us are able to get it all right. This book is for us.

In my practice, I see so many women who give everything they have to their jobs, children, husbands, and families every day, but rather than feeling that they are worthy of being put on a pedestal they feel frustrated because they are a *just few projects behind*. Simply because they are not accomplishing *everything* they wish they could, they feel like *complete failures*. And as if that weren't enough, they feel exhausted and frazzled. In my view, these women are not failures, they have simply lost sight of just how devoted they are. Their problem is not that they are achieving too little; their real issue is that they put themselves last in line, when they should be first. Why first in line? *Because everyone else in their lives depends on them.*

Are you one of these women?

If so, this chapter will provide you with tools that will allow you to do all that you want without succumbing to the heavy load that causes you to feel that you are always behind.

I've been there. For years I worked close to 120 hours a week. I was one of those obstetricians who spent the majority of the hours of labor with his patients—for hours and sometimes for days. There were very few nights that I spent a whole night at home, and my days were obviously filled with office work. In the evenings I tried to spend time with my family before leaving for the hospital for the night.

I was pushing myself every day, and I was exhausted every day.

Once I came home at three in the morning after having not slept for three nights. My body was exhausted but my mind was still racing, so I couldn't sleep. My mind was under so much stress that it *could not* cooperate with my exhausted body. I knew that I could not continue like this. On the other hand, I also knew that I could not leave my practice and family and go to an ashram in order to relax. How could I curtail this cycle of exhaustion while maintaining my health, responsibilities, and the work that I enjoyed so much?

The solution that I found is the one I will share with you here. It worked for me—and many of the women with whom I've worked over the last twenty-five years.

STRESS BASICS

Stress results from any challenge or threat, either real or perceived. The stress response is the body's activation of physiological systems—beginning with the hypothalamus area of the brain, continuing to the pituitary gland and then to the adrenal gland—that produces a hormone called cortisol, which provides us with the boost of energy necessary to escape harm. Unfortunately, chronic activation of the stress response can lead to wear and tear on your body that eventually predisposes you to disease. Research shows stress damages your cardiovascular system, elevates your blood pressure, and increases memory loss. Stress also decreases your overall immunity, increases incidence of breast cancer, back pain, headache, and hair loss.

In other words, stress is nothing to wave off or brave through. *Stress is deadly*.

On a cellular level, the overall increase of cortisol resulting from stress also promotes cell destruction. That's right; the simple act of allowing something to "get to you" causes you to *destroy cells.* This affects the way your brain works, the way your organs function, the way your skin and hair look, and whether your body aches or not. Stress immediately affects *everything.* And over the long term, stress can cause you to *look* as frazzled as it makes you *feel.* For this reason, the last thing you should do is wave off anything as "just stress."

SEEING STRESS FOR WHAT IT IS

I have always described stress as the raucous, angry crowd that encourages boxers to clobber one another to a pulp. The crowd wants conflict, not peace. The crowd wants to promote violence, bloodshed, knee-jerk responses, and angry reflexes, not thoughtful, quiet resolution. The crowd wants destruction, not well-being.

The similarities between an angry mob and your body's physiological response to stress explains why you are likely to perform poorly when you feel stress. Indeed, your ability to function physically and mentally is substantially diminished when you feel this way. This is because the fight-or-flight response is designed to have you think less and respond more in order to escape. In this moment that you feel stress, your body is diverting energy from all other systems—including your brain—to energize your ability to be physical. In one moment, you revert to a cavewoman, surrendering all of your years of evolution as a species and all of your personal years of education as a human being. In today's world of stress, this fight-or-flight response actually causes you to perform less well than you usually do. That's why it takes so much more energy and mental focus to perform as well under stress as you do when you feel calm—your overall ability to be competent is compromised. This is also the reason why you sometimes find yourself baffled as to why you could have performed so illogically under pressure—saying and doing the wrong things.

Moreover, the expenditure of energy and mental focus to perform well under stress is exhausting, and often causes you to experience greater strain, which triggers the stress response anew. Some people—and I count myself in the early days of my career in this group—live with this cycle of increased stress every day. Some women I speak to report that it's a fact of their "lifestyle" or their "career choice." In light of what you now know that stress does to you on a physiological level, doesn't that sound crazy?

Certainly this explains why being a Natural Superwoman and performing at your best requires you to manage your stress.

NEUTRALIZING STRESS THE NATURAL WAY

Many of us use our many external responsibilities as excuses for ignoring our body's needs. We allow our own equipment to experience the damage we do to our bodies and minds until we experience some measure of "system breakdown"—an injury, an illness, or an emotional breakdown. For people who pride themselves on getting a great deal done every week, this may seem counterintuitive: we take care of our jobs, children, and relationships—we say we will do *anything* for our kids—yet many of us completely fail to address our own basic needs, instead allowing ourselves to live under unpleasant conditions for weeks, months, and sometimes years. Why?

As I told you, I can answer this question quite easily. For a number of years, I got up every morning and lay down every night with the feeling that I was behind in the race. Yet I also felt that I couldn't slow down. For this reason, I found another way to manage my stress. I developed a system for calming myself down and lowering my production of cortisol. Here is the simple system I developed:

1. Identify—find the onset and source of stress.
2. Visualize—acknowledge your agitated reaction with an inner discussion and with visualization of a calm scene.
3. Breathe—take several deep and full breaths.

The following system helped me and, hopefully, it will help you in your own life:

Step One: Identify Onset

Many of the women I speak to claim that they don't feel stress creeping up on them. For this reason, the first step to reducing your stress level is actually acknowledging that it's rising in the first place. Begin by making note of your earliest physical signs of stress—you may feel your heart rate rising or a strain in the back of your neck; you feel flushed, or find that you are grinding your teeth, clenching your fists, or bouncing your legs. By taking time to see how your body reacts to a stressful situation, you will be able to cut stress off at its earliest stage.

Does it seem extreme to be so vigilant about the onset of stress? Remember, the feelings you currently identify with "everyday stress" are actually intended to help you escape life-threatening environmental stress. The next time you, your partner, or your child are being chased by a predator, I support the biological process that induces stress. Today, this type of threat is rare yet we feel the same level of stress when confronted by a boss who asks too much, a child who chronically misbehaves, a late arrival to a meeting, or the simple act of beginning the morning commute. This everyday stress you feel nonetheless taxes every one of your bodily functions. In order to prevent this, you must recognize the second your stress response begins and react to it right then. It's really deadly, it's not just part of your life, and it's not normal. Remember: stress is *not* part of living, it's part of *dying*.

At the very first moment that you identify the stress response, remind yourself of the damage it is doing to your body.

Step Two: Visualize and Have an Inner Discussion

Once you have identified how your body responds to stress and are able to pinpoint the very start of your stress response, I encourage you to work on bringing down your stress level. In my case, I use a quick technique:

Each time I feel my blood pressure rise, I visualize myself rising up, up, up to heaven, and looking down at my gorgeous wife of nearly four decades in bed with another man. As you can imagine, this gets my attention right away. It reminds me that I must immediately stop responding to a stressful situation with stress; not at the end of my day, or the end of my week. It snaps me out of my stress mode and allows me to focus on bringing down my level of tension by focusing on the techniques described in the sections that follow.

Every patient I speak to about this develops a personal visual motivation that works for her. What image would work for you? Consider imagining your skin, hair, and nails growing old at movie-fast speed, causing you to wither and leave your children behind. That's a powerful one.

Some of my patients prefer to motivate themselves with positive images. You may choose to visualize yourself on a warm beach, relaxing in the sun without a care in the world.

Whatever image you choose, practice using it while at work, on the phone, or when you are trying to concentrate on the road and your children are fighting in the backseat. Tell yourself in a soft, determined, inner voice: No. In doing so, you'll be taking a big step toward keeping that upsetting image at bay *and* literally saving your own life.

Step Three: Breathe Deeply

An easy way to remember this last step is: stress kills, but breathing heals. This is more than a slogan, it is also an accurate description of the physiological process that takes place when you inhale.

Once you have identified your stress reaction and used your personal visualization to cut it off, sit up straight, keep your shoulders low, and take a good, deep breath. Take in oxygen in a slow, even, relaxed manner. Most people who are stressed cannot inhale deeply. As they do, they jerk their shoulders up, which strains their neck and upper back muscles, causing additional physical stress and tension. Keep your shoulders down and breathe in a calm, effortless way. Expand your chest as much as you can as you breathe in. Don't worry if you cannot do all of this the first time you try; most women experiencing stress cannot follow this simple instruction.

Next, say to yourself: *I am calm. I am relaxed.*

Now hold your breath—without tension, without stress, without undue effort, for as long as you can. In doing so, you are expanding your lung capacity and learning to breathe more effectively. Are your shoulders still down? This is the point when many women unconsciously bring their shoulders to their ears. Make an effort to keep yours low and relaxed.

As soon as holding your breath becomes difficult, begin exhaling slowly through your mouth. As you exhale, you should feel your navel contracting back, back, back, until it feels as though it is about to kiss your spine. As you exhale, keep your posture straight.

If you've just tried this exercise now, ask yourself how you feel. Chances are that you feel just a bit better having taken a deep breath. That's because simply holding your breath has been shown to reduce oxidative stress and acidity in your blood—both associated with the early stages of cell and tissue destruction.

Just like that, you've curtailed cell destruction in your body. And the nice thing about this step is that you can practice it anywhere—at work, in the car, in the ladies' room. If you are with people, put your hand under your jaw and breathe silently. Focus. Practice this step often, anytime you can.

Some women reading this will try these three steps and feel relief right away. But regardless of whether you feel anything today, if you use these steps each time you feel your stress response kicking in, in a few weeks you will begin to notice that you can do more. Imagine, with three little steps you can release yourself from the stress straps that effectively restrict you from being your best self—that keep you from *soaring*.

MEASURING AND CONTROLLING STRESS WITH MEDICAL ASSISTANCE

Are my three steps enough? For those who intervene really early on, it can be. But if you're reading this chapter, chances are you are farther along the path of physiological destruction that is associated with stress.

How do you know how bad off you are? When a woman visits me at my office, a large portion of my time with her is spent assessing where she is along the path of stress-related destruction.

Beyond speaking to a patient, the best way to determine just how much damage stress has done to a woman's body is by testing her level of cortisol—the hormone her body produces when she feels stress—at various points in her day. In my office I test for cortisol levels using:

* Blood testing
* Urine testing
* Saliva testing

UNDERSTANDING STRESS BIOCHEMICALLY

* **Perfect adrenal function.** Under normal circumstances, your adrenal gland produces measured amounts of cortisol in the morning, when you are meant to be most active and productive. This supply of cortisol tapers off as the day wears on, and remains relatively low in the evening and night, when you are meant to be resting.

* **Adrenal overproduction.** When you feel any kind of stress, your adrenal gland produces cortisol to give you an immediate boost of energy that will help you escape from your predator. In such a case, you need to scramble out of harm's way in a relatively short period of time. When you experience modern living during an average workday, or over several weeks when faced with the illness of a loved one, your body continues to function at the same level of intensity for as long as your anxiety lasts. In some cases, you live a *lifestyle* of constantly running from predators. This continuously floods your body with high levels of cortisol—way more than you were designed to tolerate and far more than your adrenal gland was designed to produce. Women who produce this level of cortisol may feel constantly wired, alert, and in control. I have observed that

they tend to exercise quite a bit, despite a hectic schedule. In fact, most high-achieving women that I meet *love* this stage, because they feel that they can accomplish anything they set their minds to.

When I test the blood, saliva, or urine of women who are overproducing cortisol, I am able to see that their overall level of cortisol production is high throughout the day, rather than just in the morning.

- **Adrenal transition.** Of course, at some point, these women turn a corner. Some begin having a hard time going to sleep or *staying asleep,* because their bodies are flooded with cortisol day *and* night, contrary to the high-in-the-morning, low-in-the-evening rhythm humans were designed to enjoy. When does adrenal overproduction become adrenal transition? This depends on:

  - Your particular genetic predisposition.
  - How strong your adrenal gland is to start with.
  - How intense your stress is.
  - How long your stressful condition lasts.

  In a small group of women who happen to be exceptional sleepers, adrenal transition will not change their routine in the early stage of this process, which delays their feeling the other symptoms associated with the wear and tear on the adrenal gland. But ultimately, these symptoms catch up with these women, as well.

  When they do, all women enter the second part of the adrenal transition phase. In this phase, while you may not realize that you are exhausting yourself, you will begin to feel small cracks in your armor. You may notice that:

  - You cannot accomplish what you could previously.
  - You may feel that your mind is unfocused, and races.

- You are not as physically vigorous as you used to be. When you exercise one day, you may feel the need to take the day off on the following day.

These small setbacks may not feel like much, but they are just a taste of what is to come.

Believe it or not, most of your female coworkers and neighbors are living in adrenal transition. Despite the widespread nature of this condition, diagnosing this phase is tricky: cortisol levels in your blood, urine, and saliva may not be consistent, levels may sometimes be high and sometimes low. Moreover, a level that is high for you may not register as such when compared to the general population.

- **Adrenal exhaustion.** As you can imagine, because the adrenal gland was designed to quickly produce cortisol in occasional, short bursts, constant cortisol production ultimately leads to wear and tear that begins to make itself known. Like a battery that is slowly losing its juice, the adrenal gland eventually begins producing less and less cortisol, earlier and earlier in the day. In some cases, the adrenal gland functions like an on-and-off switch: because of its severely limited capacity, it produces cortisol for a few hours in the morning, and then completely shuts down for the rest of the day. Either way, you begin to feel fatigued. The moment you acknowledge this is when you enter adrenal exhaustion. Where you used to feel "wired" and "high" all day and night, you may now feel that you have no energy at all, even in the mornings. Other symptoms may include:

  - Exercise fatigues you, either immediately or after a certain point that would have been easy for you in the past.
  - Work exhausts you, where it may not have consistently done so before.
  - You feel exhausted at night, but your racing mind prevents you from sleeping, or sleeping well.

- Loud noises and hot or cold temperature are intolerable to you.
- Adventurous opportunities seem like too much trouble—you have no interest in packing a bag and heading out to go hiking.
- You crave sweets more than usual, in some cases at night, because there is not enough cortisol to feed your brain with sugar, and your brain cannot operate without sugar.
- You crave salt more than usual, because your adrenal gland moderates blood pressure and your adrenal gland cannot do this on its own.

This phase of stress is currently experienced by a large number of women living around you.

- **Complete adrenal depletion/Addison's disease.** Eventually, like a dying battery, the adrenal gland just peters out. In blood, urine, and saliva testing, women in this phase evidence perilously low cortisol levels. When observed using MRI imaging, the adrenal glands of women in this phase evidence a decrease in size by 50 percent.

This end stage, where the adrenal gland has only minimal reserves available, is Addison's disease, a life-threatening condition that requires immediate medical attention. Indeed, without a functioning adrenal gland, you would not survive more than forty-eight hours, even in the best-equipped emergency room.

Adrenal depletion must be treated with cortisol by an endocrinologist and is beyond the scope of this book.

OBTAINING TESTING

Because every woman reading this book falls into her own slot on a wide range of normal cortisol production, unless you're at the very end stage of complete adrenal depletion, testing for the destructive effects of stress is not cut-and-dried. The best diagnoses are based on an understanding of your personal history and how you feel every day. Did you once enjoy rock concerts and now can't stand noisy performance halls? Did you previously enjoy running and now feel wiped out by thirty minutes of brisk walking on a treadmill? Communicating with your physician about *how you feel* and *how you've changed* is important in the early stages of the stress process because by the time your blood, urine, or saliva tests show your cortisol effects, you may already be very far along.

In my practice, my recommendation for testing depends on what my patient has reported to me about how she feels and where I think that description puts her in the chain of stress events. The more tests I run, the farther along I believe my patient may be.

- **Cortisol blood test:** This test measures the level of cortisol in a patient's blood at the time the blood is taken. I generally administer this test before nine a.m. on a day when the patient is experiencing an average amount of physical and emotional stress—not the day following vacation or a day predicted to be difficult at work. Why? Between six and nine a.m. your level of cortisol should be at its highest point. As is the case with all testing, the range of normal differs between labs. The lab I use indicates that normal results range from 5 to 25, and I regard a result that is over 15 to be high, and anything under 8 to be low.

  Women who are in the adrenal transition group may yield results that are all over the map, depending on how much stress they feel at the time of their test and how long they have felt that way. For this reason, the information I get from the patient herself helps me make my ultimate decision about where this patient is on the continuum and how much help she needs.

- **Blood cortisol stimulation test.** This test was first described about forty years ago by pioneer endocrinologist Dr. William Jeffries, who applied this test to thousands of patients he followed up with for more than thirty years. Understanding his work is a must for any physician interested in understanding stress and cortisol management. Interpreting the results of Dr. Jeffries's test is complex; for this reason, the test should be administered by a physician familiar with this protocol.

- **24-hour saliva test.** While blood tests work as a spot test, providing a picture of cortisol production at the time the test is taken, the saliva test provides an example of your daily fluctuation of cortisol levels over the twenty-four hours during which the test is administered. The patient is asked to spit into four separate containers that are submitted to the lab— in the morning, at midday, in the afternoon/evening, and at night. The aim of this test is to determine whether your cortisol production is following the natural order of high cortisol in the morning and low cortisol at night, as would be evident in a woman in the perfect adrenal group.

  Women in the adrenal overproduction group will evidence high cortisol levels throughout the day and into the evening.

  Women in the adrenal exhaustion group may evidence low cortisol throughout the day, with no morning spike and two or three out of the four measurements reading abnormally low.

  As mentioned before, women in the adrenal transition group may produce results that are all over the map. Some measurements may be high, and others low. For this reason, *speaking* to these women is the best indicator of where they are.

- **Urine test.** This test provides another method for measuring the cortisol produced by your adrenal gland, but in this case it measures your total average cortisol production over twenty-four hours. Urine testing is complex and requires interpretation by a physician who has experience in treating women with adrenal disorder.

TREATING STRESS USING THE FOUR PILLARS

Mind and Mood Balance to Decrease Stress

As a physician focused on nutritional and hormonal remedies, I generally begin any treatment discussion with the diet and nutrition and hormone pillars. However, in the case of stress and adrenal challenge, any attempt at recovery must begin with the basic mind and mood relaxation steps outlined at the start of this chapter. Without arresting the genesis of the stress response, all efforts to boost nutritional or hormonal conditions are useless. Regardless into which group along the stress continuum you fall, I suggest beginning with the following:

- Use the steps for identifying, visualizing, and breathing described on page 214. Simply recognizing your stress is a reliever. But making the decision not to tolerate stress as an acceptable part of your life will help prevent future damage.

- Address the underlying causes of your stress. If you are anxious (Chapter 13), cannot sleep (Chapter 14), or if your mood is low (Chapter 12), make an effort to address these root causes.

- Reintroduce calm and relaxing activities into your life. Even if you must switch out part of an intense workout for a more relaxing breathing class or a midday walk around the neighborhood where you live and work, make short breathers part of your day.

Treatment for Group 1: Overproduction/High Cortisol

When I meet a woman who I believe is in the adrenal overproduction group, it is sometimes necessary for me to convince her that she should rethink her activity level, because she feels great. She's high on energy and likely to be thinner than ever, more alert, and able to run all day and night. She believes nothing is wrong with her.

But at the same time, that patient will express frustration about feeling stressed out and uptight. I generally point out that the benefits of being able to overproduce are related to the burdens of not being able to sleep, and feeling tense and short-tempered. My aim is to help them understand that they are taxing their adrenal glands, and that without a break, this gland will soon show signs of wear and eventually malfunction.

I recommend the following:

- **Step 1: Incorporate the Identify, Visualize, and Breathe steps.** Address the causes of stress and incorporate relaxing activities into your schedule as described above (page 214).

- **Step 2: Remove all excessive stimulants from the diet.** Do you drink many cups of coffee per day? Remember that large take-out containers of gourmet coffee may contain between three and four shots of espresso. How many of these do you consume per day? I recommend you cut down to two coffees or two shots of espresso per day. I also suggest reducing cigarette smoking and limiting use of herbal stimulants, including diet pills.

- **Step 3: Modify your diet to optimize nutrition.** Choose whole foods, prepared healthfully, or if this is not possible for you, consider supplementing the nutrients recommended in Chapter 1.

- **Step 4: Modify or add physical activity.** If you are not physically active, add light activities to your daily routine, but be sure these do not exhaust you. If you are on the other end of the spectrum and exercise quite a bit, consider my earlier recommendation to add more calming modalities, including yoga, meditation, Pilates, stretching, and tai chi to your routine.

- **Step 5: Consider supplementing your diet** with nutrients that specifically support your adrenal gland.

NUTRITIONAL SUPPLEMENTS
THAT SUPPORT THE ADRENAL GLAND

- **Vitamin B complex.** I recommend supplementing 25 to 100 mg daily, in the morning, with food. Reduce dosage if you feel agitated.

- **Vitamin B$_5$.** I recommend supplementing 50 to 200 mg daily, in the morning, with food. Reduce dosage if you feel agitated.

- **High-absorbable magnesium** (glycinate or ionic sublingual). I recommend supplementing 400 to 1,000 mg, split into two or three doses a day, taken with food. Reduce dosage if your experience loose stool.

- **Adrenal adaptogen.** Herbs that assist your adrenal gland in readapting lost adrenal sensitivity can be helpful. In women who feel a great deal of stress, the cortisol faucet is stuck in the "on" position and will only turn off once it is fully depleted. This herbal support helps your adrenal gland regain its ability to turn off when you'd like. By the same token, when you need more cortisol, adaptogen will support your adrenal gland and help it produce more in order to provide you with energy when you need it.

HORMONES THAT SUPPORT THE ADRENAL FUNCTION
Supplementing the following hormones can also help women in the adrenal overproduction group support their adrenal gland.

- **DHEA** counterbalances the negative affects of high cortisol levels and helps decrease cortisol levels as needed. DHEA also increases progesterone, allopregnenolone, and your production of endorphins. For more information on how to supplement this hormone, see Chapter 7.

- **Pregnenolone** can also be helpful in restoring proper adrenal function, but be aware that it can also produce further agitation in some women, even in low doses. For more information on how to supplement this hormone, see Chapter 8.

- **Melatonin** is extremely important to women in the adrenal overproduction group, because it can lower levels of nighttime cortisol, allowing you to increase your number of sleeping hours. This will help you avoid further adrenal deterioration. For more information on how to supplement this hormone, see Chapter 14.

- **Human growth hormone (HGH)** also helps reduce nighttime cortisol levels, just as melatonin does. It is my clinical observation that many of the women in the adrenal overproduction group who tend to overexercise actually have lower HGH levels, and I believe this group will enjoy additional benefits by correcting their relative HGH deficiency. For more information on how to supplement this hormone, see Chapter 6.

- **Progesterone** is a key hormonal tool for the treatment of women who are experiencing the effects of stress. When progesterone works well, it's ideal—it calms, helps you sleep, and reduces cravings for sugar. For more information on how to supplement this hormone, see Chapter 5.

- **Allopregnenolone** is a metabolite of progesterone, which means that progesterone is produced by the body and some of it converts into allopregnenolone. This hormone serves as women's natural form of Valium or other mood enhancer. Bioidentical allopregnenolone is not currently in wide use, but in the future it will be used as an extremely effective tool for calming women who feel anxious, allowing them to transition off other medications.

Treatment for Group 2:
Adrenal Exhaustion/Low Cortisol

When you reach the stage of adrenal exhaustion, your adrenal is no longer able to provide the energy you require for the basic human instinct of fight or flight. You feel completely exhausted by *any* physical or emotional activity. Beyond activity, even loud noises or changes in temperature are intolerable to you. Your battery is at its lowest point ever, and this affects every aspect of your life and can become life-threatening in the form of Addison's disease if it goes untreated.

Unfortunately, medicine offers very little to women who haven't yet reached the point near or at Addison's disease. In my practice, I recommend that patients follow step one through five recommended for the adrenal overproduction group (page 224) and then supplement the following:

NUTRITIONAL SUPPLEMENTS THAT SUPPORT
THE ADRENAL GLAND FOR WOMEN IN GROUP 2
(ADRENAL EXHAUSTION/LOW CORTISOL)

- **Vitamin B complex.** I recommend supplementing 25 to 100 mg daily, taken in the morning, with food. Reduce dosage if you feel agitated.

- **Vitamin B$_5$.** I recommend supplementing 50 to 200 mg daily, taken in the morning, with food. Reduce dosage if you feel agitated.

- **High-absorbable magnesium** (glycinate or ionic sublingual). I recommend supplementing 400 to 1,000 mg, split dose into two or three doses a day, taken with food. Reduce dosage if you experience loose stool.

- **Adrenal gland extract** (nonvegetarian). I also recommend supplementing this product as directed.

HORMONES THAT SUPPORT THE ADRENAL GLAND FOR WOMEN IN GROUP 2 (ADRENAL EXHAUSTION/LOW CORTISOL)

Supplementing the following hormones can also help women in the adrenal exhaustion group support their adrenal gland.

- **DHEA** may energize you and help you sustain this energy. It also acts as a mood elevator and memory enhancer, and generally compensates for the lack of cortisol in women in the adrenal exhaustion group. Supplementing DHEA allows you to regain your fight-or-flight instinct, which, in turn, allows you to do more and feel exhausted less often. For more information on how to supplement this hormone, see Chapter 7.

- **Pregnenolone** works hand in hand with DHEA in restoring proper adrenal function and your natural instinct for fight or flight. For more information on how to supplement this hormone, see Chapter 8.

- **Progesterone,** a woman's natural Valium, may be helpful if your exhaustion is also accompanied by anxiety. Note that one of the side effects of taking too much progesterone is a feeling of dizziness, which is especially problematic for women in this group, as this is a symptom of adrenal exhaustion. For this reason, supplementing progesterone must be slow and careful, to prevent supplementing too much. For more information on how to supplement this hormone, see Chapter 5.

DHEA, pregnenolone, and progesterone represent a great start for regaining energy and stamina when you are in the adrenal exhaustion group. But these three hormones are really just the first step. I highly suggest the inclusion of the following:

- **Hydrocortisol.** This bioidentical cortisol supplement is recommended as a treatment for patients with Addison's disease. However, *in much lower doses,* it is also ideal for bridging your body's need for cortisol while your adrenal gland recovers and until it can resume production.

Be sure that the dose you take is not the dose recommended for Addison's patients, because a large dose will completely shut down production of the small amount of cortisol your recovering adrenal gland is able to make. This is counterproductive to your recovery process. On the other hand, if you receive the proper dose of hydrocortisol, you may find that it changes your life practically overnight. You'll be able to return to a productive life—physically, mentally, and emotionally. Ideally, I recommend that patients take advantage of this renewed energy to address the underlying reasons—sleep, stress, anxiety, diet, activity, and emotional realities—why their adrenal glands became overused in the first place. This will slowly allow you to return to a more normal adrenal function. It's a slow process, but with commitment, it works and improves the lives of the women who embark on it.

In general, the younger you are, and the less time you have been exposed to the underlying reasons that bring about adrenal exhaustion, the more likely you are to recover your normal adrenal function and the faster this recovery will be. In my mind, "recovery" is returning to normal level of activity without requiring the use of hydrocortisol.

- **Using hydrocortisol.** In my practice, I recommend bioidentical oral hydrocortisol.

Oral hydrocortisol should be taken a half hour before meals and the activity for which you anticipate needing an extra boost of energy. Swallow with water and a mouthful of protein to avoid indigestion. If you do experience indigestion, address this with your physician, as hydrocortisol can produce ulcers in rare circumstances. Hydrocortisol works quickly, but the effects last only four to six hours.

Avoid consuming carbohydrates when you take your dose of hydrocortisol, as any type of carbohydrate—including the "good kind" of carbohydrates like salad—will decrease absorption.

I recommend supplementing 0 to 15 mg in the morning, although most of my patients take 5 to 10 mg in the morning. In the midday, I recommend supplementing 0 to 10 mg, with my average patient dose being 5 to 7.5 mg. In the evening, I recommend supplementing 0 to 5 mg, with my average patient dose being 0 to 2.5 mg.

In the beginning of your treatment, start at the low end of my dosage recommendations. If this initial dose is too high for you, you will feel agitated. This is your cue that you must begin with a lower dose.

Some women will not respond to hydrocortisol treatment even at the highest dose. This may be because they have Addison's disease and require a far higher dose under the supervision of an endocrinologist. Alternatively, some women may have a variety of viral diseases, Lyme disease, significant excess heavy metals in their system, or some other condition that prevents them from responding to this treatment.

At midday, take a moment to reassess the challenges that lie ahead in your afternoon. Generally, women need less cortisol in the afternoon, but if your day will include mental or emotional stress at work, or you have a workout scheduled, you may need to take a dose equal or greater to your morning dose.

Your evening dose of hydrocortisol is a different story. Remember, naturally, your cortisol production should go down in the evening in order to allow you to sleep. Because a hydrocortisol supplement lasts for four to six hours, the afternoon dose may be all you need. If you find that you are not sleeping, reduce or eliminate your evening dose.

However, if you find that returning home two to three hours before you plan to go to sleep you crave sweets and feel tired, despite having a whole evening of work or chores you must accomplish before you can head to bed, definitely consider a supplement of hydrocortisol. Remember, a craving for sweets is one of the prime characteristics of cortisol deficiency. Your brain effectively runs on sugar, and needs more of it during times of stress. Cortisol assists the sugar in reaching the brain, curbing your craving for outside sources.

By the same token, if you plan to go out for an evening of activities and you feel tired, consider boosting your energy level with a dose of hydrocortisol.

An Alert Regarding Hydrocortisol Treatment

- **Don't overtreat** and therefore abuse hydrocortisol in order to engage in activities that are too much for you. Even if you have historically enjoyed strenuous hikes, you may not be able to now—you may have to settle for lighter ones. Although you may have been an accomplished runner prior to your adrenal exhaustion, your running may have inadvertently thrown you into your adrenal crisis, so consider that you may now have to be a brisk walker.

In my personal battle with adrenal exhaustion, I managed to recover from my first bout by using the program outlined here. Eventually, I was even able to stop using hydrocortisol. Then, five years later, when I was no longer putting in the all-night shifts as an obstetrician, I took a morning walk while on vacation. As I watched other people running past me, I thought, "Maybe I'm strong enough to start running again?" I restarted my running program right then and there, and within one week, I had regressed right back into adrenal exhaustion. The difference was that, this time, I was older and my body had a harder time recovering. I realized that maybe I should consider that running was no longer for me. I wasn't that eighteen-year-old paratrooper in the Israeli army. I also wasn't an ob-gyn who worked 120 hours a week. I felt good, but to continue doing so without consistently sustaining injuries, I had to face the fact that I do need to supplement some hydrocortisol, and that I must set realistic goals. Now, on our yearly visits to the same beach, I speed-walk hand in hand with my beautiful wife, without the injuries and fatigue I suffered earlier, and I, well, feel *great*.

- **Don't undertreat.** Let's assume you are compliant and not overusing your cortisol. There will nonetheless be days when you cannot predict how you will respond to your activities. Following physical activity you may begin to feel flu-like symptoms. Or a meeting at work may cause you to feel physically, mentally, and emotionally exhausted. If this happens, immediately supplement 2.5 mg of hydrocortisol. It's crucial to avoid a challenge to your adrenal gland at any cost, as this trauma will delay your recovery.

- **When healing from injury.** Be conscious of the fact that you must decrease your dose of hydrocortisol as you heal. As you begin to feel better, your first response should be to decrease your dose, rather than increase your challenges. For example, if you take hydrocortisol to walk three miles, which you could not do without supplementing hydrocortisol, once you accomplish your goal of walking three miles, cut down your dose rather than endeavoring to *run* those three miles. Remember, this hydrocortisol is a remedy; it's not meant to be a lifestyle.

- **When you have colds and flu.** Colds and flu can be the most difficult challenges for women with adrenal exhaustion. Women suffering from this condition tend to get colds and flu easily and recover from these ailments very, very slowly. Personally, I try to do everything I can to avoid contracting common colds and yearly flu. I make a point of washing my hands whenever I enter my house or office, I take additional supplements before, and every four hours during and after flying, or when I am around people who are obviously sick, and try to be extra mindful of how I feel in winter.

When you have a cold or the flu, you must stop *all* physical activity and decrease emotional stress as much as you can. Any activities that are not essential should be rescheduled. Take the maximum amount of hydrocortisol that you would take on a day during which you are active, despite the fact that you are not. Believe me, your body needs it. This may eliminate the flu on arrival or *significantly* decrease its duration. When you feel that you have recovered, as you gradually decrease your dose, gradually increase your activity. Do not jump back into your normally active schedule—build up, as you would a vitamin program.

In the last six months, I managed to decrease my morning dose from 15 to 7.5 mg, although I still take an additional 2.5 mg at midday. Very rarely, I take an additional 2.5 mg in the evening. When I have a cold or the flu or feel that I'm coming down with one, I immediately stop my activity and jump back into my full dose of 10 to 15 mg in the morning, around six a.m., 5 mg around midday, and 2.5 to 5 mg around 8 p.m.

• **After surgery or accident.** The recovery of people with adrenal deficiency from surgery, invasive procedure, or injury is usually very slow. Before your procedure or before receiving treatment of any kind, it is your responsibility to inform your doctor and anesthesiologist of your average daily dose of hydrocortisol. Usually, your doctor and anesthesiologist will provide your adrenal gland with additional support during surgery and treatment, and may even give you additional support as a follow-up. Do not use a hydrocortisol supplement if you receive an alternative support from your doctors, but consider reintroducing your program once this other support program is completed.

The treatment of adrenal exhaustion with hydrocortisol should be administered by a physician who is familiar with this treatment modality, not with a nutritionist or a health-care provider who is not an M.D. (medical doctor) or D.O. (doctor of osteopathy).

Note: Melatonin and HGH should not be used by women in the adrenal exhaustion group, as these women cannot afford to further lower their cortisol. Many of the side effects of low cortisol are similar to those with low HGH. Taking HGH while in adrenal exhaustion may cause you to enter into an Addisonian crisis. Women interested in supplementing HGH should have their adrenal gland evaluated thoroughly.

GROUND RULES FOR GROUPS 1 AND 2 IN RECOVERY

- **Avoid physical activity that makes you feel fatigued** immediately thereafter or within a few hours.

- **Immediately acknowledge** if you are experiencing a period of increased physical, emotional or mental stress, or sleeplessness for more than a few nights. Do not ignore these conditions. Instead, apply all of the steps described—Identify, Visualize, and Breathe—to restore a sense of calm in your life. You cannot afford not to.

Treatment for Group 3: Adrenal Transition

The treatment for women in the adrenal transition group is far less defined than that for women in the overproduction and exhaustion groups. This is because women in this group present symptoms from both other groups. For this reason, treatment for this group must be individually tailored to the symptoms described by the patient. If you feel that you are in this group, I encourage you to work with your physician to identify your symptoms and address them individually using the recommendations provided for the overproduction and exhaustion groups.

Jean's Story

Jean, forty, has three children, and is in relatively good shape. But as she sat in my office, her body language indicated that she was not relaxed. I noted that she didn't move much during our conversation, and seemed glued to her seat. She didn't smile and she tended to clench her teeth.

When we spoke, she explained that she had recently begun to feel exhausted after her usual morning four-mile run. And because she juggles her job, her three children, and her relationship, at the end of the day she feels too tired to look after all of the things that running a household requires. Despite this, when she lays her head down on her pillow, she often finds that she cannot fall asleep.

Because of this, even though she is a relatively conscientious eater, Jean has lately discovered that she needs more than her usual one cup of coffee in order to stay alert. She now requires a cup before her run, a cup after, and two or three more during the first half of her day.

When I asked Jane to breathe in front of me, despite her weekly yoga and Pilates, she couldn't. Her breathing was short and shallow. And with each breath, she jerked her shoulders up, further tensing her neck. When I checked Jean's blood tests, I noted that her adrenal hormones, DHEA and pregnenolone, were within normal limits but nonetheless lower than expected for her age. Her twenty-four-hour urine test indicated that her cortisol levels were normal in the morning, but she was low on metabolites. Her saliva test indicated that her cortisol did not peak in the morning, but *did* peak at night. No wonder she was tired in the morning and couldn't sleep when she laid her head down.

This scenario is typical of someone in the transitional group, but is by no means the only story. Yours will be unique, but will have the following characteristics in common:

You are trying to do the best that you can with the energy you have.

You want to be active.

(continued)

You want to eat well.

You want to spend time with your kids.

You want to apply yourself to your professional endeavors.

You want to do what must be done around the house.

You also want to connect with your partner.

If you're in the transitional group, you're probably having trouble accomplishing all of these goals, and without intervention, you'll find that you have less and less energy to do what you must.

For Jean, I recommended the following:

- Until recovery, decrease morning physical activity. Rather than running, consider walking.
- Incorporate the Identify, Visualize, and Breathe steps described on pages 214 to 216. Apply this approach to every minute, day and night—in the car, while making food, when lying in bed and not sleeping.
- Address anxiety, as recommended in Chapter 13.
- Address sleep disorder, as recommended in Chapter 14.
- Optimize vitamins and minerals, and supplement adaptogen.
- Apply a combination of treatments from the adrenal overproduction and exhaustion groups that address Jean's individual symptoms, including supplement adrenal support, DHEA, pregnenolone, in the morning, and 5 mg of hydrocortisol and melatonin and HGH to sleep.

Jean, like all women in the adrenal transitional group, required treatment modalities taken from both the high cortisol and low cortisol groups. A physician with experience in cortisol treatment can help you identify your patterns and recommend individualized treatment protocols for morning and evening.

In general, so many of us live with a certain degree of adrenal deficiency that goes untreated because we have not reached the bottom—Addison's disease. Addressing this deficiency could significantly improve your outlook on life, and the earlier you do something about it, the more benefit you will enjoy.

12 • Depression

Answer the following questions to find out if you may be suffering from depression:

Do you feel that you sleep too much? Or, are you having trouble sleeping?

Do you avoid going out or socializing?

Do you find that things, activities, or people that used to please you no longer do?

Do you wear less makeup than you used to?

Are you less concerned about the way you look, in general?

If you've gained weight, are you unconcerned with this change in weight?

If you are single, have you avoided going out on dates recently?

If you are partnered, do you find that you have lost interest in your partner for no specific reason?

Have you lost or increased your appetite?

Have you stopped exercising, or are you exercising less?

Has anyone commented that you are less smiley than usual? Less communicative?

Have you been less interested in longtime hobbies?

Do you find yourself avoiding confrontations? Giving up during conflicts?

Have you found that you cry more easily?

Do you find that you are less motivated than you used to be?

If you relate to a number of these conditions, you may be experiencing some measure of depression and could benefit from taking steps to elevate your mood.

DEPRESSION BASICS

The only good thing about being depressed is that you are not the only one—in North America alone there are millions of depressed women to keep you company. Globally, the numbers are even higher. Today, depression affects girls and women much earlier than it ever has and becomes more common as women grow older. Millions of women treat their depression with prescription antidepressant medications—and for some, these medications are lifesaving—while millions of others use supplements, counseling, exercise, activities, prayer, or chanting to stave off their feelings of sadness. With all of these treatments for depression, North Americans should be the happiest, least depressed people on the planet, yet as a group we are not.

My feeling is that depression still plagues us as a culture because we do not address this condition from a nutritional, hormonal, and mental perspective. In the pages that follow, you will find four pillar tools that I currently use in my practice to help my patients eliminate or reduce depression, and live happier, more balanced lives.

USING THE FOUR PILLARS TO CONTROL DEPRESSION

Depression is serious business. In your fight against depression, you must arm your body with the best possible tools in order to give it a chance to recover. At the end of the day, what you provide your body may be just as important as medication, forced socializing, or counseling.

IDEAL DIET TO CONTROL DEPRESSION

What does your diet have to do with a disease like depression? Quite a bit. Although you may already know about how refined sugars affect mood, did you know that populations whose diet focuses on eating whole foods in moderate portions actually experience lower incidence of depression? Conversely, the fewer nutrients and more toxins a given population consumes, the higher their incidence of depression. In addition, a diet rich in whole, fresh foods and low in refined carbohydrates and processed sugars will help your body fight the side effects of depression, including obsessive-compulsive disorder (OCD), insomnia, anxiety, and attention deficiency disorders (ADD/ADHD).

More specifically, the following foods contain nutrients that are uniquely helpful in supporting your body's fight against depression:

- **High-quality, high-cocoa-content chocolate** is high in antioxidants and in magnesium, a supplement with significant mood-elevating properties. To enjoy the benefits of cocoa without the drawbacks of sugar, I recommend melting high-cocoa-content unsweetened chocolate with stevia, a natural sweetener, berries, and almond flour (or pulverized almonds), spreading it on a cookie sheet, and refrigerating it for two hours. Enjoy a moderate number of pieces after your evening meal.

- **Low-mercury *wild* seafood** that is high in omega-3 fatty acids is especially supportive of mood balance. I recommend four to six ounces several times a week.

- **Leafy green vegetables** such as kale, spinach, and collard greens are high in the whole range of vitamin B complex, a family of nutrients known to support mood balance. I recommend consuming significantly more vegetables than current meal programs call for—two to three vegetables a week. I recommend increasing your consumption to a full pound of vegetables *a day* if possible.

DO YOU GET A SWEET TOOTH WHEN YOU'RE BLUE?

Many women who are depressed are also sugarholics. In addition to being a pro-oxidant that promotes inflammation, sugar can directly exacerbate mood disorders. Reducing your sugar intake is paramount to managing your overall mood balance. If you find that you eat a great deal of refined sugar, it is unlikely that simply hearing this advice will be enough to curb this habit. Consider transitioning your current consumption by making better choices. Choose fruit or beverages that contain sweeteners such as stevia, which does not increase the level of sugar in your blood when it is consumed. If you crave ice cream or another dessert, choose one with high-quality, natural ingredients, or a home-

(continued)

made chocolate dessert that does not contain preservatives. Of course, in all your choices, be sure to make a point of consuming less this week than last week, until you eat fewer than three desserts or other foods with refined sugars per week.

Unfortunately, not one of us eats as well as we'd like. For this reason, when a patient visits me in my office, I often recommend she supplement vitamin B complex, magnesium, fish oil, and other nutrients to address deficiencies in her diet. In addition, I run blood testing to determine her levels of folic acid, vitamin B_{12}, and vitamin D. For patients wishing to balance mood, these nutrients should be on the high end of the range considered normal or be supplemented one at a time, as described in the following section.

NUTRITIONAL SUPPLEMENTS TO CONTROL DEPRESSION

Combating depression nutritionally begins with supplementing the nutrients recommended for increasing serotonin and dopamine levels (page 247). Additionally, the following nutritional supplements specifically help control depression. Add each of these to your daily intake one at a time, with two weeks between the start of one and the addition of a second.

Why Add Supplements One at a Time?

If you've ever visited a psychopharmacologist for antidepressant medication, you may have noticed that he or she will prescribe a series of medications one at a time. You may begin with an antidepressant that increases serotonin, and then if this isn't effective, your doctor may add something to increase dopamine, and then after that he or she may add a third medication that increases serotonin and norepinephrine. This same approach is recommended for treatment of depression with nutritional supplements.

Why is the treatment of depression seemingly so haphazard? The fact is that the human brain is complex and not yet fully understood. This is especially true of brain chemistry. Medical science does not currently have the ability to measure baseline neurotransmitter levels, and therefore cannot accurately predict both what a patient is low on and what the "ideal" *individual* level for that patient is. Current urine testing is simply not predictive enough. For this reason, physicians use the "wait and see" approach—they prescribe a medication and wait for the patient to describe how it makes them feel. If one medication is not ideal, doctors try another, based on the feedback he or she receives. I believe that future urine, saliva, and brain activity testing will be more helpful in understanding what patients need and how this need can be efficiently met. In order to receive the most benefit from today's medications, it is vital that you communicate with your physician and remain an active advocate for your *individualized* course of treatment. In other words, you are the ultimate determinant of whether you feel better.

The following nutrients should be added in the order in which they appear:

- **Saint-John's-wort.** I begin with this nutrient because it's able to increase serotonin, dopamine, and norepinephrine. In addition to increasing serotonin levels, Saint-John's-wort also increases the levels of other neurotransmitters, which makes it especially effective for treating mood and anxiety disorders.

Although a much-publicized study published in the *Journal of the American Medical Association* (*JAMA*) found Saint-John's-wort ineffective in treating mood, it has since been understood that the dosage used for this study was far too low to yield results. In fact, this same study also found the prescription antidepressant medication Zoloft to be ineffective at elevating mood. By contrast, multiple studies have illustrated that Saint-John's-wort is as effective as, or is significantly more effective than, 20 mg of Prozac. In my clinical experience, Saint-John's-wort is an efficient herbal tool that is also easy to use and rarely produces side effects.

Saint-John's-wort is an herb, but does not naturally occur in common human foods. You may supplement 300 mg, three times daily, with or without food. If you don't feel positive effects after one week, double your dose *over the course of a week*, building up slowly until you reach 600 mg, three times daily.

- **5-hydroxytryptophan (5-HTP).** My second treatment protocol is 5-HTP. Depending on initial response, I either add 5-HTP to the Saint-John's-wort or advise my patient to take 5-HTP instead of Saint-John's-wort. I like this supplement because it increases serotonin levels, and in doing so calms, relaxes, and reduces appetite. 5-HTP is able to cross the brain barrier, where it converts to serotonin. In other words, 5-HTP increases serotonin levels by actually *making* serotonin. Because of this, high levels of 5-HTP provide many of the benefits associated with serotonin, including a significant decrease of depression and anxiety, while also curbing food cravings.

5-HTP is not present in significant amounts in a typical diet. And although our bodies produce 5-HTP from L-tryptophan, eating foods that contain L-tryptophan does not significantly increase our 5-HTP levels. For this reason, elevating 5-HTP levels generally requires taking natural supplements.

To supplement 5-HTP, I suggest taking 50 to 300 mg, up to three times daily. If you are taking too much, you will feel sleepy or experience a runny stool due to an overproduction of serotonin in your gastro-intestinal tract. Like with all natural substances, some women will have paradoxical, or opposite-than-expected results. Although I have seen it rarely in my practice, a study has indicated that in some cases 5-HTP can increase cortisol, and therefore make women feel more anxious than relaxed. If you feel anxious after taking 5-HTP, discontinue use and refer to one of the other supplements recommended.

- **L-tryptophan.** The presence of this amino acid in turkey is the substance that causes you to feel so relaxed after Thanksgiving dinner. This same calming benefit is available when you supplement L-tryptophan. Once you identify your ideal food or supplement dosage of L-tryptophan, you will be able to raise your serotonin levels without feeling sleepy.

  L-tryptophan provides other mind and mood benefits beyond its ultimate conversion to serotonin. The conversion process itself requires oxygen and prompts us to take deeper, more fruitful breaths—essential to promoting relaxation and every other biological function that requires adequate oxygenation. In other words, simply breathing deeply and mindfully allows you to increase your serotonin levels. For further discussion on how full breathing contributes to our biochemical process, see the Chapter 11.

Side effects and L-tryptophan In the past, L-tryptophan enjoyed extreme popularity as an herbal supplement, until it was discovered that the inventory of the largest Japanese producer had become tainted by another substance. A number of consumers experienced side effects not previously associated with L-tryptophan and it was largely abandoned as a supplement. Since then, the source of the contamination was discovered and corrected. Today, L-tryptophan is extracted from milk and safe vegetarian sources.

(continued)

In general, I find that L-tryptophan is more effective with sleep disorders than depression, although I have found that in a few women, L-tryptophan is the *most* effective substance I can recommend for depression. In other words, as with all natural substances, the benefits you can expect are highly individual.

L-tryptophan is found in lean meats, poultry and egg whites, dairy products, soy products such as soy milk, tofu, and soybeans, nuts (hazelnuts, peanuts), seeds (sesame and sunflower), and legumes (lentils and chickpeas), but must be supplemented in order to enjoy the calming benefits described here.

You may supplement 500 to 2,000 mg during the day and another 500 to 3,000 mg at night, with or without food. Decrease your dose if you feel sleepy or if your mouth begins to feel dry.

- **SAMe.** I turn to this nutrient last because the cost of SAMe is relatively high. SAMe is an incredible longevity supplement that can improve and protect liver function, in addition to providing anticancer protection. It can also be an efficient antidepressant, rarely with side effects.

When you visit the health food store, you may find two types of SAMe available—one version costs 50 percent more and is twice as effective. My recommendation is that you purchase the more expensive variety if possible. SAMe must be taken during daylight hours only. It is not effective if taken after the sun has set. Take 200 mg on an empty stomach (thirty minutes before food or two hours after food), twice a day. Increase your dosage every ten days to two weeks to a maximum dose of 800 mg, twice daily.

THE ROLE OF DOPAMINE
IN CONTROLLING DEPRESSION

Often if you feel depressed, optimizing your level of dopamine can be helpful.

NUTRITIONAL SUPPLEMENTS
TO INCREASE DOPAMINE

The natural sources listed below may help you do this. I recommend beginning with both L-theanine and casein tryptic hydrolysate, and adding fish oil (DHEA/EPA) and thyrosine if the first set of supplements is not sufficient. If this is still not sufficient, you may add L-arginine, Saint-John's-wort, ginkgo biloba, and pygnogenol, as instructed.

- **L-theanine.** This amino acid is able to cross the brain barrier and can therefore directly increase dopamine levels. L-theanine is found in green tea, with decaffeinated green tea recommended, and is regularly used as a mood enhancer in Japan, but must be supplemented in order to enjoy the benefits described here. You may supplement 100 to 600 mg daily, with or without food. Reduce levels if you feel sleepy.

- **Casein tryptic hydrolysate.** This new supplement is derived from milk extract and enhances dopamine levels. In my practice, I recommend a combination of casein tryptic hydrolysate and L-theanine called Brain Nutrients, and suggest patients take two to three capsules, two to four times daily, with or without food.

- **Fish oil (DHA/EPA).** Fish oil, and in particular the DHA portion, promotes dopamine levels by causing dopamine neurotransmitter receptors to become more sensitive, increasing the ability of dopamine and serotonin to bind to their receptors, and reducing levels of norepinephrine, an agitating neurotransmitter.

  Adequate levels of DHA/EPA are found in *wild* fish. In order to limit exposure to mercury, choose types of fish that are smaller, and are therefore more likely to contain lower levels of mercury. Look for DHA/EPA in capsule or liquid form that indicates that it is derived from low mercury sources. Supplement 1,000 to 2,000 mg, twice daily, with food. It must be supplemented in order to enjoy the benefits described here.

- **Tyrosine.** This amino acid is an essential precursor to the production of dopamine. Does this mean that ample doses of tyrosine will guarantee a sufficient amount of dopamine? Unfortunately, no. Our bodies only allow a certain amount of tyrosine to convert to dopamine, at any given time. In my clinical experience, I have found that increasing tyrosine levels helps combat the fatigue that can be a side effect of foods and supplements that increase GABA and serotonin levels.

  Tyrosine is found in lean meats, seafood, tofu, egg whites, skim milk, yogurt, green beans, and seaweed, but must be supplemented in order to enjoy the benefits described here. You may supplement 500 to 1,000 mg, twice daily, with or without food.

- **L-arginine, Saint-John's-wort, ginkgo biloba, and pygnogenol.** These supplements have been found to elevate dopamine levels and may be additionally supplemented individually, or in combination. Use as directed by the packaging of the supplement you purchase.

Adding the nutrients described above while taking antidepressant medication or attempting to replace your antidepressant medication with these supplements must be done under the direct supervision of a physician who is familiar with this process.

HORMONE SUPPLEMENTS TO CONTROL DEPRESSION

Hormones are the most powerful tools at your body's disposal for controlling depression. Unfortunately, rather than using bioidentical versions of these hormones as a first line of treatment, if at all, most women I speak to recount that they only hear about this treatment option when all other pharmacology fails. Some patients are never even given the option.

Having worked with bioidentical hormones and nutrients as a first line of treatment for depression for more than twenty-five years, I believe that if women were offered hormone treatment first, they would not experience the high failure rate currently seen with the use of pharmacological drugs alone.

- **Estrogen.** In my experience, bioidentical estrogen is the most ideal antidepressant medication available to women because:

  - It directly promotes the effects of serotonin, dopamine, and nor-epinephrine.
  - It acts as a strong monoamine oxidase (MAO) inhibitor, maintaining your supply of serotonin and dopamine in their work centers.
  - It serves as a GABA stimulator.

Estrogen may be safely used as an antidepressant by women at any age, not just those who are menopausal. Taking estrogen for any reason requires individualized dosing information available in Chapter 4.

- **Progesterone.** Progesterone can help combat depression by:

  - Serving as a mild MAO inhibitor.
  - Enhancing the effect of estrogen on serotonin.
  - Serving as a strong GABA stimulator.

  In my practice, I find that low doses of progesterone can be effective in treating milder cases of depression. However, if a patient is relatively older and her symptoms are severe, supplementing progesterone may block her estrogen function and inadvertently enhance the severity of her depression. For this reason, I do not recommend progesterone as the first course of treatment to manage significant depression.

  Taking progesterone for any reason requires individualized dosing information available in Chapter 5.

- **Thyroid.** Every woman with severe thyroid deficiency feels depressed. However, many women who fall into the broad normal thyroid production range but who are nonetheless producing too little thyroid for their individual needs may also experience some measure of depression. It is common for this group to be nonresponsive to antidepressant medication because their treatment must first address their suboptimal thyroid levels. This phenomenon is becoming better known in the psychopharmacological community, and thyroid supplement is often recommended to nonresponsive cases. I feel that if you have a mild thyroid deficiency, simply supplementing thyroid before you take antidepressant medication may resolve both your thyroid deficiency and your depression altogether.

Amanda's Story

Five-foot-three-inch Amanda is sixteen. She was brought into my office by her mom, who explained that her daughter had been a happy, well-adjusted teenager, a good student, and a strong athlete. At age fifteen, Amanda began experiencing irregular periods, depression, and weight gain of about five pounds. Her family doctor recommended a common treatment—he prescribed birth control pills to resolve Amanda's irregular periods and a relatively low dose of antidepressant medication. Within six months, she had gained close to twenty pounds and felt more depressed than ever. She even stopped exercising.

When I spoke with Amanda, I asked her to describe her symptoms before and after her initial treatment. The symptoms she experienced prior to her birth control treatment evidenced a mild thyroid deficiency; she reported that she awoke with less energy than before, had gained weight, noticed some hair loss, occasionally felt constipated, and no longer perspired as quickly when she engaged in physical activity. To this list I added her irregular periods, also associated with thyroid deficiency. Despite all this, Amanda's thyroid levels were never checked.

Unfortunately, the birth control treatment recommended to Amanda significantly aggravated her thyroid deficiency. Why? Birth control pills increase levels of a protein called sex-binding globulin, which decrease the already suboptimal amount of thyroid available to patients like Amanda. In exacerbating her thyroid condition, the birth control pills caused her to gain more weight, lose more hair and energy, feel more constipated, and made her feel even more depressed than before taking antidepressant medication.

Many women with thyroid deficiency do not respond to antidepressant medication. In Amanda's case, she wasn't responding to her second treatment medication—the antidepressants—because her thyroid levels were low, and brought down even lower by her birth control

(continued)

pill treatment, exacerbating her low thyroid symptoms, including her depression.

Amanda's irregular periods and lack of interest in physical activity were not resolved by her birth control pill treatment. Because of the way oral contraceptives work, they further suppressed her natural ovarian function, increasing her level of sex-binding globulin, dramatically *decreasing* her available testosterone levels, and affecting her interest in physical activity. For more information on how birth control pills affect natural hormonal function, see pages 188 and 290.

Her blood work confirmed all this, so I recommended that Amanda cease using birth control pills and begin a low dose of a natural thyroid supplement increased every two weeks, while gradually decreasing her antidepressant medication. In three months, Amanda had lost most of the twenty-five pounds she had gained; she had one normal menstrual cycle, and her mood and energy improved, while her constipation decreased. She stopped losing hair, and she seemed to be on her way to a full recovery without antidepressant medication.

- **DHEA.** This hormone produces an antidepressive effect in women of all ages. Taking DHEA for any reason requires individualized dosing information, available in Chapter 7. In particular, see the section on depression within this chapter.

- **Melatonin.** Melatonin has an antidepressive effect and should be considered for depressed women with sleep disorders. Taking melatonin for any reason requires individualized dosing information, available in the section on melatonin found in Chapter 14.

- **Human growth hormone (HGH).** Treatment with HGH is not a traditional antidepressant tool, but in my practice I have found that HGH deficiency causes women to lose their oomph, or what I call "life's vibration." Taking HGH for any reason requires individualized dosing information, available in Chapter 6. In particular, see the section on depression within this chapter.

- **Cortisol.** Women with adrenal exhaustion and significant fatigue due to low cortisol levels are often also depressed. In my experience, when you address adrenal exhaustion with cortisol supplement, a feeling of well-being improves and depression may resolve. For more information on how adrenal activity can affect mood, including treatment recommendations, see Chapter 11.

Depression is a serious illness not to be taken lightly. This section is not meant to encourage anyone to abandon her antidepressant medication, or even to replace her medication with any of the recommendations described above. For some women, conventional psychopharmacological medication is a lifesaving tool. In my experience, many women find the suggestions provided here to be more helpful overall. No woman should make the switch from antidepressant medications to these hormone supplements without the direct supervision of a medical professional who has experience in this process.

Barbara's Story

Barbara, forty-one, is a stay-at-home mom with two children and a stable relationship. During an office visit, she explained that while she had always felt somewhat low throughout the month, and actually depressed premenstrually, in the last year, this normal depression had become much worse. In this same time frame, she had gained ten pounds, had lost more hair than usual, had more indigestion and dry skin than usual, and occasionally felt anxious and experienced periodic insomnia. Barbara said she couldn't live this way.

Her previous doctor had prescribed several types of antidepressants, but these made her feel numb and left her with neither sexual drive nor

(continued)

response. Her gynecologist recommended a treatment with birth control pills, but these only caused her to feel more depressed. Barbara was desperate.

In our first meeting, I observed that Barbara had suffered from lifelong PMS, which seemed to be getting worse with time. She had many of the subjective signs of thyroid deficiency, including hair loss, constipation, dry skin, and weight gain, and had episodes of anxiety associated with insomnia.

Barbara's blood workup revealed that she was neither menopausal or even premenopausal, although she had a B complex and magnesium deficiency, which contributed to her depression, anxiety, and constipation. In addition, she suffered from a mild thyroid deficiency, which contributed to her PMS, depression, hair loss, and constipation. Her naturally relatively low estrogen and progesterone levels contributed to her lifelong history of PMS and depression, and she had an increase in nighttime cortisol and low DHEA levels, which contributed to her high anxiety and insomnia.

I decided to treat her in a two-stage program. First, I focused on addressing her insomnia, depression, and anxiety. I recommended that she supplement magnesium, vitamin B complex, vitamin B_6, and the amino acid taurine, all combined in a proprietary formula that I use in my practice called TranCalm (page 261). I also added melatonin to this group in order to reduce Barbara's nighttime cortisol to help her sleep and elevate her mood.

Additionally, I recommended that she treat her depression with a combination of estrogen and 5-HTP. Barbara and I discussed how to adjust her estrogen dose depending on where she was in her cycle and how she felt on a given day. Her supplement of 5-HTP helped reduce her depression, and also helped her decrease food cravings and ultimately return to her previous weight.

Three months later, Barbara reported that her mood had significantly improved, and that she hadn't felt this good in many years. She still complained of hair loss, unresolved constipation, only moderate weight loss, and the emergence of some fluid retention.

In the second step of her treatment, I focused on these remaining symptoms, including her borderline thyroid deficiency. I recommended that she supplement natural thyroid to address her mood and reduce her weight, hair loss, and constipation. I also suggested the addition of bioidentical progesterone to balance her estrogen and correct her minor water retention. The addition of these two hormones allowed Barbara to resolve her remaining symptoms within three months. On her next office visit, she reported that she was supplementing much less estrogen than she had originally required and felt that she was back, only better than ever!

ACTIVITY MAINTENANCE TO CONTROL DEPRESSION

Activity and body movement can help to elevate your mood. Consider the following in conjunction with your nutritional and hormonal efforts.

- **Get out of bed.** Always begin your day by getting out of bed. It is not acceptable for any woman who wants to feel better to spend the day in bed and indoors.

- **Posture—let it speak for you.** The way you carry yourself says a great deal about how you feel. A slouched upper back, a concave chest, and a chin that points toward the ground communicate a sense of defeat. Conversely, standing up straight, stomach held tight and chin high, communicates to others—and to yourself—that you are ready to face anything, that you are in control of the challenges of today and ready to face those of tomorrow. So even if you are not feeling well, and you are sure that the whole world is conspiring against you, get up, stand straight, and begin your activity with a look of strength. In doing so, you make a statement that you refuse to be controlled by whatever depresses or upsets you, and that you prefer to determine how you feel.

- **Take care of your looks.** Looking good is feeling good. Take a shower and start your day fresh. Put on a colorful outfit that you've been complimented on before. Often, we forget how much better we feel after bathing and receiving a few compliments on a flattering wardrobe choice.

- **Try light exercise.** I have yet to meet any woman or man who increased physical activity in a moderate and responsible way and became more depressed. Any physical activity, at any level and at any time, is a great first step to elevating mood. More important, some exercise is better than no exercise. If you feel that you are not in the mood to exercise, just take a walk.

  On the other hand, do not overexercise. Doing so may leave you feeling more exhausted the following day. Small amounts of exercise are far more sustainable.

- **Be social.** If you want to win the war against depression, you cannot allow yourself to become disconnected from your lifelines. The farther you get from friends, family, and coworkers, the more you will sink into feeling blue. Consider putting "Be social" on your daily to-do list. Even if visiting with others is the last thing you feel like doing, it really is the best thing for you. Are all your friends committed to others tonight? Be inadvertently social: go to a sushi bar or a restaurant with a communal table where you are forced to interact with others. And once you're out, represent yourself well. Look your best, even if you don't care to. Challenge yourself to speak to four people, regardless of how briefly. You'll find that no matter how strange it feels, your overall condition will improve more than if you had stayed at home.

- **Address underlying mind and mood.** As with any other challenge addressed in this book, acknowledge and address the underlying issues that contribute to your depression—lack of sleep, emotional concerns, strain from a difficult work situation—do not underestimate how powerful these energy drains can be. In nearly every case, these impediments must be resolved or removed in order for you to have the energy to move forward and feel better.

13 • Anxiety

QUICK QUIZ

Answer the following questions to find out if you may benefit from reducing your anxiety level:

Do you feel that you are short-tempered or impatient, or more so than you used to be?

Do you find that your mind races?

Have you recently started smoking or increased the number of cigarettes you smoke?

Do you find that you are drinking more coffee and caffeinated beverages?

Do you grind your teeth? Bite your nails?

Do you have trouble sitting still? Do you bounce your leg? Do you pace?

Have you been told by others that you are abrasive? Have others taken issue with your behavior?

Do you find that you are not connecting with people, that everyone is annoying you?

Do you find yourself raising your voice more than you used to?

Have you experienced panic attacks? Do you feel frustrated by small things?

Do you have trouble catching your breath? Or, do you find that, in general, it is hard for you to take a deep breath?

Do your fingers tingle? Do you find that you are scratching or picking at your face? Your cuticles?

Have you noticed that you have difficulty falling asleep?

Are you speaking more quickly?

Do you feel annoyed if people don't understand you or if you have to repeat yourself?

If you recognize yourself in a number of these, then you are experiencing some measure of anxiety.

ANXIETY BASICS

Today, more of us are anxious than ever before. And just as living with daily stress has become acceptable, living with many of the awkward physical manifestations of anxiety—hair loss, irritability, impatience, and binge eating—has somehow become acceptable, too. Many men and women slowly become more and more unpleasant to be around yet assume the way they feel is normal.

In women, anxiety becomes even more pronounced in times of hormonal transition: after the birth of a child in connection with postpartum depression, as a first sign of estrogen decline in the days prior to their monthly menstrual cycle, and in perimenopause and menopause. During these times, when symptoms of mild anxiety become more severe, it is not uncommon for women to experience panic attacks with many of the same signs as heart attack—the onset of anxiety can be *that* sudden and terrifying.

Isn't it amazing that our culture of "acceptable stress" causes some women to feel that that they are imminently dying or that they are going crazy? How can this be acceptable? Clearly, it is not.

Biochemically, anxiety promotes destructive processes that include the overproduction of glutamate, epinephrine, norepinephrine, and cortisol, while limiting the production of much-needed GABA and serotonin.

Being a Natural Superwoman means rejecting anything that others may regard as normal but that is not optimal for *you*—inside and out. Rather than shrugging off pebbles in your shoe that slow you down and make you less efficient, I encourage you to address the core issues that keep you from focusing on your individual excellence, however you may choose to define that for yourself.

DOES ANXIETY MOTIVATE?

Although a sense of urgency is helpful for "getting off your duff" and accomplishing something you've been putting off, any task will be more effectively and more quickly completed with a clear head.

USING THE FOUR PILLARS TO CONTROL ANXIETY

Every pillar remedy that helps relieve stress (Chapter 11) will also help alleviate anxiety. Eating whole foods in moderate portion sizes while managing your intake of stimulants will arm your body with the nutritional tools it requires to help you manage the way you feel. In addition, as I will describe below, the nutritional supplements such as magnesium, vitamin

B complex and vitamin B$_6$, and fish oil (DHA/EPA) recommended for promoting GABA and serotonin and controlling your production of glutamate will also help you to control anxiety.

Nutritional Supplements to Increase GABA

The following natural nutritional supplements increase GABA and help reduce anxiety. As with pharmaceutical antianxiety medications, some will help elevate your mood at varying doses, and others may not affect you unless taken in combination with others. Finding the right mix of natural supplements will be a highly individualized process.

If you feel anxious, I suggest that you begin by supplementing the first set of supplements—L-theanine and taurine—and see how you feel once you identify your highest-tolerated dose. If this combination is not sufficient, I recommend *additionally supplementing* the second set—vitamin B$_6$ and magnesium. If you are still feeling anxious, I recommend adding the third group—inositol and N-acetyl cysteine (NAC)—and after this group, L-glutamine and GABA supplement, until your anxiety subsides. In my practice I use two blends—TranCalm, a formula that combines vitamin B$_6$, magnesium, taurine, and NAC, and also ZEN, a combination of L-theanine and GABA supplement. In my experience, these blends allow me to cut the time required to find the ideal combination for my patients. I generally recommend that patients begin with TranCalm and take one to four capsules, two to four times daily, with or without food. If this is not sufficient, I suggest additionally supplementing ZEN, and take one to four capsules, two to three times daily, with or without food. If a patient is extremely agitated, I recommend that she start with both.

L-theanine and Taurine

- **L-theanine.** This tea extract is able to cross the brain barrier and make you feel more calm by directly increasing your GABA levels—all without a prescription. L-theanine additionally calms by reducing the stimulating effect of caffeine. Yet another benefit of L-theanine is that it protects neurons, the nerve cells that transmit information in the brain and nervous system, from decreasing when they are exposed to free radicals. Many of my patients choose to supplement L-theanine and find it calms them without compromising their vitality and energy. L-theanine is found in tea, with decaffeinated tea recommended. You may supplement 200 to 800 mg daily, split into two or three doses, with or without food.

• **Taurine.** This inhibitory, or calming, amino acid increases GABA's effect, decreasing stress and anxiety. Taurine is found in lean animal proteins, seaweed, nuts, legumes (lentil and soybeans), onions, garlic, cabbage, turnips, and Brussels sprouts, but it must be supplemented in order to enjoy the calming, antianxiety benefits described here.

To supplement taurine, you may take 1,000 to 5,000 mg daily, with food. Taurine is nonaddictive but has the benefits of many medications that are habit forming. However, like many other natural supplements, you won't feel its effects immediately. I recommend that you begin at the highest dose you can tolerate and wait to see how it makes you feel over time. If the amount you take is too high, you'll know right away, because you'll likely feel fatigued. Simply reduce your dosage by 1,000 mg until you regain your energy. Once you find your highest-tolerated dose and begin to enjoy the benefits in a predictable way, you may find that you can reduce your dose as you begin to feel generally more calm. On the other hand, you can always increase your daily dose on any given day when you anticipate having to do something that challenges your positive mood—a difficult day at work, a confrontation, or an emotionally challenging family gathering. In rare instances, Taurine will not be effective in elevating your mood, and may even cause you to feel depressed. If this occurs, stop supplementing immediately.

Vitamin B$_6$ and Magnesium

- **Vitamin B$_6$.** This vitamin increases GABA by ensuring that other B complex vitamins function as intended and assists in alleviating mood and nervous system function. Although B$_6$ is found in a variety of foods, including lean meats and poultry, fish, egg whites, small legumes (such as lentils and soybeans), cabbage, and watermelon, it must be supplemented in order to enjoy the calming, antianxiety benefits described here. To supplement B$_6$, you may take 100 to 300 mg daily, with food. B$_6$ should always be taken with 25 to 50 mg of a comprehensive B complex vitamin.

- **Highly absorbable magnesium (glycinate or sublingual).** Any program focused on increasing GABA should include a highly absorbable form of magnesium, nature's form of Valium. Beyond relaxing you, the combination of vitamin B$_6$ and magnesium provides significant support to countless systems in your body, including your hormonal system. Because this combination is so simple and safe, it is often overlooked as an obvious remedy for mind and mood balance. Although found in low-mercury fish such as halibut, dry roasted nuts (i.e., almonds and cashews), legumes such as soybeans and black-eyed peas, and leafy green vegetables such as spinach, magnesium must be supplemented in order to enjoy the calming, antianxiety benefits described here.

Look for magnesium glycinate in pill form or sublingual ionic magnesium. Ideal dosage is 400 to 1,000 mg daily, with food, beginning with the lower dose and increasing by 100 mg daily. Reduce your dosage if you experience a soft stool or diarrhea or if you feel *too* calm for your taste. Note that like other natural remedies, magnesium requires supplementing at your personal maximum for six to eight weeks or more before you feel its benefits.

Inositol and N-Acetyl Cysteine (NAC)

- **Inositol.** In addition to supporting liver function, high doses of this B complex vitamin also elevates GABA levels, making it especially good as a natural antidepressant and sleeping aid. Although inositol is produced by the body and is also found in nuts, legumes (including chickpeas), cantaloupe, and citrus fruits (excluding lemons), it must be supplemented in order to enjoy the calming, antianxiety benefits described here. Consuming a lot of caffeine may result in an inositol deficiency, which is associated with irritability, mood swings, skin eruptions, hair loss, and constipation. I generally advise patients who feel anxious to limit or avoid food or drink that stimulates them, as coffee does.

  To supplement inositol, take 2 grams in the morning and 4 to 10 grams at night, daily, with or without food.

- **N-acetyl cysteine (NAC).** This combination of three amino acids enhances GABA production, in addition to providing gentle liver support. NAC's various amino acid building blocks are found in high-protein foods, including meats and dairy products. The combination must be supplemented in order to enjoy the benefits of all three of these amino acids at levels that can help alleviate anxiety. I recommend taking 500 to 1,000 mg, twice daily, with or without food.

L-glutamine and GABA Supplement

- **L-glutamine.** This amino acid supports liver function and the gastrointestinal tract, enhances muscular energy and function, and is a precursor to the production of GABA. L-glutamine is found in lean protein, egg whites and other dairy protein, wheat germ and oats, but must be supplemented in order to enjoy the calming, antianxiety benefits described here. To supplement L-glutamine, I suggest taking 1,000 to 4,000 mg in the morning and at night, with or without food.

- **GABA supplement.** I include a direct GABA supplement on this list as a good muscle relaxant, even though it does not cross the brain barrier, and therefore cannot increase GABA where it is needed to improve mood. GABA is not naturally occurring in foods, and may be supplemented by taking 500 to 2,000 mg, two to three times daily, with or without food.

HORMONE SUPPLEMENTS TO INCREASE GABA

If you have a more dire condition, tools that provide a more immediate effect, such as hormone treatments, may help. I always begin with progesterone and estrogen, and add each of the hormones that follow in the order they are presented here.

- **Progesterone** is the hormone that most positively affects GABA levels. This is likely the result of progesterone's conversion to allopregnenolone. The amount of progesterone and, in turn, allopregnenolone that you have in your system makes a big difference in the way GABA functions and how you feel. The use of progesterone is highly individual; see Chapter 5 for dosage information.

- **Estrogen** is incredibly helpful in decreasing anxiety because it increases serotonin levels and promotes GABA function. The use of estrogen is highly individual; see Chapter 4 for dosage information.

- **DHEA, melatonin, and HGH** may help reduce anxiety by helping to decrease cortisol levels, one of the culprits responsible for causing us to feel anxious. For information on the individualized use of these hormones, see Chapters 6, 7, and 14.

Similarly, activities such as moderate exercise and socializing, both of which promote the efficacy of serotonin, also provide relief from anxiety. In fact, many women who identify themselves as stressed and anxious report that exercise is one of the few things—chemical or otherwise—that helps them relax.

NUTRITIONAL SUPPLEMENTS THAT DECREASE GLUTAMATE

Balancing your glutamate production is another key to reducing anxiety. Calming supplements that increase GABA also protect against the effects of glutamate. For this reason, many of the same nutrients are recommended below. Begin by supplementing the first two listed—magnesium and vitamin B_6—together. If this combination is not sufficient, I suggest adding the N-acetyl cysteine (NAC) and fish oil. If you still feel anxious, add SAMe, followed by L-theanine and taurine.

In my practice, I recommend that patients begin with TranCalm, a formula that combines vitamin B_6, magnesium, taurine, and NAC, and suggest one to four capsules, two to four times daily, with or without food. If this does not suffice, I recommend that my patients supplement SAMe.

- **High-absorbable magnesium (i.e., magnesium glycinate or ionic sublingual magnesium).** Magnesium reduces the production of glutamate under ischemic conditions where the body lacks enough oxygen, such as stress, physical trauma, arterial sclerosis, and brain clots.

  Additionally, magnesium behaves like a noncompetitive NMDA (N-methyl-D-aspartic acid) -receptor antagonist, meaning that it prevents NMDA from attaching to the glutamate receptors and beginning the degeneration processes associated with Alzheimer's.

Magnesium-rich foods include low-mercury fish such as halibut, dry roasted nuts (i.e., almonds and cashews), legumes such as soybeans and black-eyed peas, and leafy green vegetables such as spinach, but magnesium must be supplemented to enjoy the benefits addressed here.

Look for magnesium glycinate in pill form or sublingual ionic magnesium. Ideal dosage is 400 to 1,000 mg daily, with food, beginning with the lower dose and increasing by 100 mg daily. Reduce your dosage if you experience a soft stool or diarrhea or if you feel too calm for your taste. Note that, like other natural remedies, feeling the benefits of magnesium requires supplementing at your personal maximum for six to eight weeks or more.

- **Vitamin B$_6$.** Proper levels of vitamin B$_6$ decrease glutamate. B$_6$ deficiency increases neuronal irritability and lowers the seizure threshold. B$_6$ rich foods include lean meats and poultry, fish, egg whites, small legumes (such as lentils and soybeans), cabbage, and watermelon, although B$_6$ must be supplemented in order to enjoy the benefits described here.

  You may take 100 to 300 mg daily, with food. Vitamin B$_6$ should always be taken with 25 to 50 mg of a comprehensive B complex vitamin.

- **N-acetyl cysteine (NAC).** NAC is a glutamate inhibitor, which decreases glutamate by replacing it with cysteine. The three combined amino acids that make up NAC do not naturally occur in foods. NAC's various amino acid building blocks are found in high-protein foods, including meats and dairy products. You may supplement 500 to 1,000 mg, twice daily, with or without food.

- **Fish oil (DHA/EPA).** These fish oil nutrients protect the brain against the cell destruction affects of NMDA (N-methyl-D-aspartic acid) by decreasing brain hyperexcitability (i.e., migraine, seizure), including agitation and stress. Adequate levels of DHA/EPA are found in wild fish. In order to limit exposure to mercury, choose types of fish that are smaller, and are therefore more likely to contain lower levels of mercury. In order to enjoy the benefits described here, I recommend that you nonetheless supplement fish oil. Look for DHA/EPA in capsule or liquid form that indicates that it is derived from low mercury sources. I recommend you supplement 1,000 to 2,000 mg, twice daily, with food.

- **SAMe (S-adenosyl-L-methionine).** This natural nutrient is found in nearly every living cell in the body. SAMe makes adenosine, a substance that decreases glutamate. SAMe does not occur naturally in human foods and must be supplemented to enjoy the benefits described here. You may supplement 200 to 800 mg, twice daily, between meals. Take another 200 to 800 mg dose before nightfall.

- **L-theanine.** This vitamin crosses the brain barrier and decreases glutamate. L-theanine is also found in green tea, with decaffeinated green tea recommended. You may supplement 100 to 600 mg daily, with food. If you've taken more than is ideal for your body, you may feel more calm than you'd like to be.

- **Taurine.** This amino acid rescues brain neurons from the toxic effects of high levels of glutamate. Taurine is found in lean animal proteins, seaweed, nuts and legumes (lentil and soybeans), onions, garlic, cabbage, turnips, and Brussels sprouts, but must be supplemented in order to enjoy the benefits described here. You may supplement 1,000 to 5,000 mg daily, with food.

A more thorough discussion of how the hormone, mind and mood, and activity maintenance pillars assist in remedying specific mind and mood conditions follows in the discussion of each condition.

Michelle's Story

Michelle, thirty-eight, is a single trial lawyer with no children. As a partner in a successful law firm, she typically works twelve hours a day—even longer in the last three months, because of a challenging trial. She generally ends her days with two hours at the gym, which makes her feel great, but reports that her work schedule was so intense during the last two months of the trial she was not able to work out regularly.

Michelle came to see me after she experienced severe chest pains and heart palpitations one morning during her last menstrual period. Her coworkers called 911 and she was whisked away, but at the hospital, Michelle was diagnosed with a panic attack and discharged with a prescription for the antianxiety medication Xanax.

When we met, my first impression was that Michelle was thin, looked relatively nervous, gasped for air during speech, and held her shoulders high, rather than in a lower, relaxed fashion. I don't think she smiled the whole time we sat together. She reported that her diet was poor, and dominated by fast food containing unfavorable carbohydrates and poor-quality protein.

Michelle, and many others, are the women for whom I write this book. Michelle and women in her situation—whether they work in an office or in the home—give one hundred percent to their challenges. But in doing so, they forget about maintaining their four pillars, maintaining *themselves*.

I recommended a full chemical, metabolic, nutritional, and hormonal workup for Michelle. As expected, her results revealed the following:

- Michelle was hypoglycemic. Her high-carbohydrate, high-sugar, fast-food diet had caused her to develop a sugar sensitivity. The day before her panic attack, she had consumed mainly unfavorable carbohydrates, with little or no protein or essential fats. Her hypoglycemia significantly contributed to her panic attack.

(continued)

- A twenty-four-hour saliva test indicated high cortisol levels throughout the day and into the night. Michelle was always "on." Another woman in her situation would have had problems sleeping, and experienced anxiety much earlier, but I guessed that in Michelle's case, her hours of exhaustive gym time allowed her to manage her high-cortisol-related anxiety. Once Michelle's trial work forced her to curb her gym visits, this Band-Aid was no longer available to her.

- Her level of estrogen production had a natural tendency to dip lower than usual just before and at the start of her cycle. A sudden drop in estrogen can often lead to a panic attack, as it does in postpartum depression. This was yet another contributor to Michelle's attack in the early part of her cycle.

- Michelle's fast-food-heavy diet also caused her to have significant vitamin, mineral, and amino acid deficiency.

- The stressful year had depleted her DHEA and pregnenolone levels. When these two hormones are depleted, production doesn't simply return to normal when we relax.

Altogether, Michelle's circumstances were a disaster waiting to happen. Beyond my interest in explaining what got Michelle into her situation, which must be addressed and corrected to avoid a repeat episode, I also want you to understand that undoing the damage caused by this one-sided lifestyle cannot happen overnight. I recommended the following course of treatment:

As an immediate measure, I focused on increasing Michelle's GABA levels and controlling her levels of glutamate. I recommended high doses of both L-theanine, to help Michelle relax without sedation, and fish oil, as she did not care for seafood and was not consuming any other sources of essential fatty acids as part of her daily diet.

Once Michelle's immediate anxiety was under control and she had gradually tapered off her antianxiety medication, I encouraged her to begin addressing her high cortisol level and hypoglycemia as described in Chapter 11 and the section on sugar sensitivity in Chapter 12. I also suggested that she begin supplementing DHEA and pregnenolone to replenish what her body would take time to start producing again.

Michelle surprised me. She followed all of my advice regarding changing her diet. Because of her relatively by young age and willingness to consider my recommendations, her cortisol levels measured normally in a twenty-four-hour saliva test, and her hypoglycemia had corrected. In order to balance the demanding nature of her job, Michelle had replaced her two hours of intense workouts with an hour of conventional gym time and an hour of yoga or other relaxation class. Additionally, she reported that she has changed her attitude about heading to work; she no longer feels that she is going into battle, and tries to be mindful about enjoying the time she spends doing the things she enjoys in her job.

One year later, Michelle's supplement program had been streamlined significantly, and she was taking only these nutritional supplements:

- A multivitamin with high levels of magnesium, vitamin B complex, and vitamin B_6. In my practice, I use a proprietary multivitamin called Women's Longevity Formula, which contains high-quality sources for these and other essential nutrients.
- Fish oil (EPA/DHA), 2,000 mg, taken twice daily.
- DHEA, 15 mg, taken with breakfast.
- Pregnenolone, 150 mg, taken with breakfast.

Today, Michelle continues to work on managing her stress, exercising in a useful but realistic fashion, and fueling her body with foods that will allow her to maintain her demanding schedule without causing damage to her body.

14 • Sleep and Insomnia

QUICK QUIZ

Answer the following questions to find out if you need to improve the quality or quantity of your sleep:

Do you wake up in the morning and feel that you are not well rested?

Do you find that you have stopped dreaming?

Are your dreams less frequent?

Do you find that you are sleeping less soundly than before? Do small noises wake you up now, when they did not in the past?

Do you find that you must read or watch television in order to fall asleep, when you did not have to in the past?

Do you find that you need to sleep less than you used to? Are you nonetheless able to function well?

Do you find that you now wake up at night, when you did not before? Is it hard for you to fall back to sleep?

Do you wake at night with a racing pulse? Feeling hot? Perspiring?

Do you find that although your body feels exhausted, your mind does not allow you to fall asleep?

Do you have difficulty falling asleep in general?

If you identify with one or more of the conditions mentioned above, the tools described in this chapter may help you enjoy better-quality sleep. And you're not alone. Turn on the television and you'll see commercials educating you about sleep medications and their associated sleep disorders. These are not public service announcements; these ads exist because a great number of people have trouble sleeping and the pharmaceutical industry has responded with proposed remedies.

SLEEP DISORDER AND INSOMNIA BASICS

When you sleep, you restore your mental function by giving your body and brain a break from the challenges of the day. Medically, insomnia is defined as any subjective report of insufficient or nonrestorative sleep deficiency, in spite of an adequate opportunity to sleep.

This means that even though you give yourself a chance to sleep—by including the proper bed, lighting, quiet, and time—either you cannot sleep or, even if you fall asleep, you nonetheless wake up in the morning and feel that you did not sleep enough.

Insomnia is a serious and widespread condition. About 10 to 15 percent of the American population suffer from chronic insomnia, and 25 to 35 percent from occasional insomnia. Today, physicians report that younger and younger patients—even small children—complain of being unable to sleep or sleep well. And as we grow older, the incidence and significance of poor sleep increases. Interestingly, insomnia afflicts women more frequently, and far more frequently as they age.

More and more women report that they do not sleep well and wake feeling less than well rested, in spite of the fact that there is more awareness than ever about the importance of sleep and more prescription sleep medications, sleep clinics, "sleep expert" physicians, and an overall rise in consumption of over-the-counter sleep aids, natural or otherwise.

When a patient comes to see me about poor sleep, I explain that when the human body fails to perform this essential restorative function, the reasons are always complex and generally connected to the neglect of the body's four pillar needs.

CAUSES OF SLEEP DISORDERS AND INSOMNIA

This chapter does not address insomnia resulting from a specific condition that prevents you from falling asleep—back pain, postsurgical pain, and so on. This chapter also does not cover the problems of people who do not get as much sleep as they need because they believe they don't have time to do so. My hope is that this second group will read this chapter, understand the benefits of sleep, and then make it a priority. As a former obstetrician who spent nearly three decades sleeping zero to five hours a night as a consequence of having the privilege of witnessing the intoxicating miracle of childbirth at all hours, I should be the last one to preach about making sleep a priority. Regardless, I will tell you that my body shows evidence of every hour that I missed, and that I reg larly joke that in my next life, I will insist on sleeping seven hours a night.

If sleep is so important, why would our bodies deprive us of it? Most often, insomnia stems from a neglect of the four pillars:

- **Nutritional neglect.** Sleep is impaired by a neurotransmitter imbalance, amino acid deficiency, vitamin and mineral deficiency, and an excessive intake of calcium.

- **Neurotransmitter imbalance.** Physiologically, insomnia results from excess levels of glutamate, and too-low levels of neurotransmitters GABA, dopamine, and serotonin. The mechanism that helps you transition from a stage of alertness to one of sleep is compromised by this neurotransmitter imbalance.
- **Amino acid deficiency.** Amino acids inositol, L-tryptophan, taurine, L-arginine, and L-tyrosine improve the balance of the neurotransmitter levels and may decrease your level of systemic stress, allowing you to sleep.
- **Vitamin and mineral deficiency.** Magnesium, zinc, vitamin B$_6$ and B complex, and N-acetyl cysteine (NAC) are all essential to stress management, hormone balance, and neurotransmitter balance, and can therefore generally help you fall asleep and feel more well rested.

- **Mind and mood neglect.** Depression and stress are the two culprits that compromise sleep and sleep quality.

  - **Depression.** Women who suffer from depression experience a higher incidence of insomnia. One condition exacerbates the other.
  - **Stress.** When you feel stress—whether professional, emotional, or otherwise—your body envisions impending death by a predator, severe environmental stress, or hunger. In situations when your life is threatened in this way, your body would not *allow* you to sleep and succumb to a predator while unaware, it prefers that you stay awake and vigilant to preserve your own life. This is why, in spite of the fact that you may feel exhausted, if you are under a lot of stress, your racing mind may not allow you to sleep or sleep deeply. It is also the reason you may find yourself awaking and feeling agitated after only a few hours of sleep.

- **Activity neglect.** Lack of physical activity is also associated with insomnia. This is especially true for women under stress who often use excessive physical activity as a sleep aid—they can get to sleep only if they exhaust themselves.

- **Hormonal imbalance.** Hormone deficiencies and imbalance play a significant role in women's inability to sleep. Specifically, a deficiency of estrogen, progesterone, allopregnenolone, HGH, DHEA, and melatonin and an excess of cortisol must be addressed in order to restore proper sleep patterns.

PHYSIOLOGICAL CONSEQUENCES OF LACK OF SLEEP

Do you think it's all right to go without sleep for extended periods during high-performance times? Think again. When you don't sleep, the inability to rest takes a major toll on your brain and body. The results can be devastating, including:

- Epidemiological studies show that abnormal sleep patterns correlate to **lower life expectancy.**

- A third to one-half of insomniacs suffer from **mood disorders.**

- Sleep disorders also increase incidents of **cardiovascular disease** and **related death.**

- Sleep deficiency may **bring on** and **enhance depression.** In my clinical experience treating postpartum depression for nearly thirty years, sleep deprivation can often trigger and exacerbate "baby blues," postpartum depression and even postpartum psychosis, which together affect 80 percent of new mothers to some degree.

- Insomnia can increase stress and anxiety, two conditions that also enhance insomnia.

RESOLVING INSOMNIA

The average healthy Natural Superwoman must sleep between seven and eight hours every night. Some women may feel that they need more than eight or fewer than seven, but in fact this may be an indication that they have underlying hormonal deficiencies. For example, women who need more than eight hours of sleep may have a thyroid or HGH deficiency. Similarly, women who need fewer than seven hours may be overproducing cortisol. If you find that you haven't been able to get as much sleep as you need lately, do not ignore your condition. Sleep disorders can flare up quickly, wreaking havoc on your life almost immediately, and the longer you don't sleep, the more difficult it is to correct your condition. If you are not getting enough sleep, consider the following steps for improving your sleep habits:

- **Lower lights at night.** Keeping lights bright into the night prevents your body from producing melatonin and preparing you for sleep in the hours before you go to bed.

- **Lower the noise at night.** A lowered noise level provides your brain with less stimulation, making it more likely to start the process of rest.

- **Shut off the television** at least an hour before you attempt to go to sleep.

- **Decrease use of stimulants after four p.m.** This includes coffee and caffeinated tea.

- **Increase exposure to light during the day.** Interestingly, this promotes your production of melatonin at night.

- **Wind down at night.** Begin breathing and relaxation techniques in the afternoon and early evening to begin relaxing yourself in anticipation of sleep.

- **Don't provoke your brain at night.** Do not watch suspenseful, emotional, or thought-provoking educational programming at night. If you do watch television, choose light and funny shows.

- **Expend excess energy, if needed.** If you find your mind is racing in the evening, and you feel energetic, take a fast walk around the block. If you have very little energy, but your mind is still racing, take a slower walk.

- **Keep lights off once you go to bed.** Do not turn lights on if you awake during the night to visit the bathroom.

- **Don't give up.** Chase away thoughts. Don't allow them to control you. Visualize yourself sleeping well and tell yourself, "I am relaxed and calm. I am falling asleep."

- **If you wake up in the middle of the night,** breathe deeply and resume your visualization and breathing techniques.

In addition to these steps at bedtime, address your insomnia through each of the four pillars.

MIND AND MOOD BALANCE TO IMPROVE SLEEP

Immediately address the issues that can aggravate sleep: stress, depression, anxiety, and panic. If you don't, regardless of other techniques of lifestyle modifications, you will not sleep. Taking a pill that suppresses anxiety or decreases depression will not resolve the root of your problem—you'll simply be masking the symptoms and their consequences. Be proactive in your care and insist on getting to the heart of the matter.

DIET AND NUTRITION TO IMPROVE SLEEP

Eating healthfully prepared whole foods will support your hormonal balance and your adrenal function, as well. Look for foods high in magnesium, such as halibut, almonds, cashews, and spinach, and vitamin B complex, such as leafy green vegetables, nuts, and legumes.

Amino acids, found in animal protein sources, will help improve your neurotransmitter balance. I encourage my meat-eating patients to consume lean turkey, and for those who prefer not to eat meat, I recommend consuming moderate amounts of dairy. Both turkey and dairy contain high levels of the amino acid tryptophan. I advise my patients not to take calcium supplements, as this mineral depletes women's magnesium levels, maintenance of which is important for relaxing the body and promoting sleep.

NUTRITIONAL SUPPLEMENTS TO IMPROVE SLEEP

If you find that your diet does not provide all the nutrients you require in order to help you sleep or improve your sleep, consider supplementing nutrients that increase the neurotransmitter GABA and decrease glutamate (Chapter 13). If your insomnia is associated with stress and high levels of cortisol, supplement those nutrients that decrease cortisol outlined in Chapter 11. In addition, consider supplementing the following:

- **Taurine.** Taurine is a popular supplement that promotes a sense of relaxation. I recommend supplementing 1,000 to 2,000 mg daily before sleep, with or without food, and another 1,000 to 2,000 mg to help you get back to sleep if you wake up at night. For more information, see the taurine section in the discussion of GABA (page 262).

- **L-tryptophan.** I recommend taking L-tryptophan with taurine because while taurine simply calms, L-tryptophan produces a hypnotic effect. Consider supplementing 500 to 3,000 mg daily before sleep, with or without food. Begin with a 500 mg dose and increase every third day by 500 mg, as needed. If you wake up at night, take half of the dose that you took to fall asleep in the first place. For more information on L-tryptophan, see the discussion of this supplement in the section on serotonin (page 205).

- **Vitamin B$_6$ and magnesium.** I recommend supplementing vitamin B$_6$ and magnesium to relax and ease anxious thoughts. For dosage information and instructions, see the section on vitamin B$_6$ and magnesium in the discussion of GABA (Chapter 13).

- **Inositol.** Women suffering from depression who have trouble sleeping may respond to this amino acid over other treatments. I recommend supplementing 6,000 to 10,000 mg daily, before sleep, with or without food.

- **Valerian root extract.** This herb promotes sleep by increasing serotonin and GABA. Use as directed by the label on the product you purchase.

HORMONE BALANCE TO IMPROVE SLEEP

Studies on the connection between insomnia and hormonal balance conclude that both estrogen and progesterone should be considered as a first line of defense against insomnia. This supports my twenty-year clinical experience with thousands of women who successfully used estrogen and progesterone to restore their ideal sleep patterns. More often than I could count, happy patients reported they finally have their sleep back. In my experience, both estrogen and progesterone help women:

- Fall asleep.
- Stay asleep.
- Sleep more deeply.
- Dream.
- Awake feeling more rested.

Below, I more fully discuss the various forms of estrogen, progesterone, and other hormones that play a role in helping restore ideal sleep patterns.

- **Estrogen.** Insomnia is one of the clarion calls of estrogen deficiency. In younger women, this occurs premenstrually and menstrually when estrogen levels drop cyclically, or throughout the month with women who have naturally lower levels of estrogen and in young women who take birth control pills.

  Insomnia also plagues women seven to ten years before menopause, when women's levels of estrogen begin to drop. For these women, insomnia becomes progressively worse the closer they get to menopause.

  If your insomnia relates to estrogen decline, supplementing bioidentical estrogen provides a safe and nonaddictive alternative to prescription sleep medication. For more information, see the section on improving sleep in Chapter 4.

- **Estriol (E3).** Some women are unable to sleep simply because their night sweats are keeping them up. Estriol, one of the three forms of estrogen, provides a simple and safe remedy for eliminating night sweats and helping women enjoy better quality sleep. For more information, see the section on estrogen and sleep in Chapter 4.

- **Progesterone.** Progesterone can be a gift to women who suffer from insomnia. It not only allows women to sleep, it can also be helpful with complications such as sleep apnea, in both men and women. For treatment of sleep disorders, I find that creams are less effective than capsules and sublingual drops. Follow the maximum dosage recommendations in Chapter 5 and increase the dose until you are able to sleep. Decrease the dose if you experience opposite-than-expected results or if you feel sleepy and dizzy during your waking hours.

- **Human growth hormone (HGH).** Although I do not turn to HGH as a first tool in helping patients get to sleep, I find that growth hormone can provide the missing link for women who are not able to sleep using other methods. I believe that HGH works because it provides a general feeling of well-being, because it energizes women throughout the day and, if used before sleep, it decreases cortisol levels at night, allowing women to relax enough to fall asleep. For more information, see Chapter 6.

- **DHEA.** Like growth hormone, DHEA may help decrease cortisol levels at night, and may therefore help women who cannot sleep because they are agitated. DHEA must be taken in small doses and increased slowly. As with any natural supplement, it may result in an opposite-than-desired response, meaning an exhausted woman may feel more alert and energized when she should be feeling relaxed and sleepy. Discontinue use if this or any other undesirable side effect occurs and does not resolve by lowering your dose. For more information, see Chapter 7.

- **Melatonin.** This hormone is found throughout the natural world, in one-celled organisms, plants, fungi, and in most vertebrates, including humans. Melatonin production in humans is controlled by the area of your brain that also controls higher brain function, and is partially governed by whether and when your environment becomes light or dark. Melatonin is your body's chronological pacemaker: it informs your body and brain about the time of the day and year. Its hormone is also produced in your retina, gastrointestinal tract, skin, bone marrow, and your lymphocytes, a type of white blood cell. Your melatonin production peaks at puberty and then decreases throughout your life, which contributes to older people having to sleep far less than younger people.

WHY MELATONIN IS SO IMPORTANT FOR YOU

Melatonin is charged with a number of key functions necessary to good sleep and general good health.

- **Melatonin is a free-radical scavenger.** It acts as a powerful antioxidant that prevents free-radical damage.

- **Melatonin alleviates depression by improving thyroid function.**

- **Melatonin decreases anxiety.**

- **Melatonin may help repair ulcers.** In ulcerative colitis, a disease that affects the gut, melatonin repairs damage to the mucosal, or inner layer, of your gut. Melatonin heals esophageal ulcers created by medications such as Fosamax and Boniva, often prescribed for osteoporosis. I do not prescribe these medications in my practice. Melatonin also heals duodenal ulcers found in the area that food enters once it leaves the stomach.

Melatonin provides the following additional benefits:

- **Melatonin helps treat tinnitus.** Three mg of melatonin reduces tinnitus, and helps women who cannot sleep because of the ringing in their ears.

- **Melatonin helps alleviate hypertension (high blood pressure).** Three mg of melatonin at night helps decrease blood pressure in hypertensive women.

- **Melatonin promotes healthy blood platelets** by increasing platelet production and lengthening platelet life span.

- **Melatonin helps in relieving neuron-degenerative diseases such as ALS, Alzheimer's, and restless leg syndrome.** Melatonin assists in fighting these conditions by reducing free-radical formation in the mitochondria, your cells' energy centers.

- **Melatonin improves immunity.** In addition to serving as a powerful antioxidant that controls free-radical formation, melatonin boosts and improves your immune system.

- **Melatonin supports the cardiovascular system.** Melatonin has been shown to reduce cholesterol levels and decrease brain vascular damage.

- **Melatonin decreases migraines.** Women with lower levels of melatonin are more likely to suffer from cluster headaches and conventional migraines, two conditions that compromise sleep time and quality.

- **Melatonin protects the liver.** Melatonin increases glutathione formation, which may prevent liver toxicity.

- **Melatonin protects the kidneys.** Through its anti-inflammatory activity, melatonin protects the kidneys from the damage caused by infection.

- **Melatonin improves and resolves dry-eye syndrome.**

- **Melatonin protects against diabetes.** Melatonin's role as an antioxidant helps combat the damaging effects of high blood sugar.

- **Melatonin protects against osteoporosis** by enhancing the effect of estrogen in the bones.

- **Melatonin protects against cancer.** Melatonin inhibits the proliferation of various cancerous tumors and prevents them from metastasizing. Melatonin also increases the efficacy of chemotherapy and decreases its side effects. Moreover, in numerous studies on terminal cancer patients who have not responded to conventional treatments, melatonin was found to provide the following overall health benefits:

  - Helps cancer patients sleep
  - Improves patients' overall mood, including making them feel less anxious
  - Has a strong anti-inflammatory effect
  - Improves platelet production, function, and longevity
  - Acts as a strong antioxidant in the lipid (fat) and aqueous (liquid) tissue
  - Acts as a strong free-radical antagonist in the mitochondria, the energy generators of cells
  - Increases immunity, glutathione, and liver protection

- **Melatonin prevents breast cancer.** Melatonin acts as a natural aromatase inhibitor, and in doing so, decreases the incidence of breast cancer. When combined with vitamin D_3, melatonin increases the release of a natural chemical called TGF (transforming growth factor) Beta 1, which may reduce the growth of breast cancer. I recommend supplementing melatonin in relatively high doses, ranging from 10 to 20 mg, as part of the nutritional supplement program for any patient with a family history of breast cancer.

- **Melatonin supports your hormonal system.** When melatonin is given in adequate doses, it is able to reverse the decline or rise of hormonal function associated with aging. In postmenopausal women, melatonin suppresses the rise of luteinizing hormone (LH), one of the markers of menopause. In my clinical experience, melatonin also suppresses follicular-stimulating hormone (FSH) in perimenopausal and menopausal women. The increase of FSH and LH is the first sign of decreased ovarian function and an aging hormonal system.

Finally, six-month treatment with melatonin changes the gonadotropin, a stimulating hormone that converts into a number of other hormones essential to brain function, increasing these hormones to levels on par with those found in much younger women.

- **Melatonin as contraceptive.** In fact, *very* high doses of melatonin (75 mg)—far in excess of what the casual user would consume—have contraceptive effects.

- **Melatonin promotes longevity.** Treatment with melatonin significantly improves the brain's response to inflammation—the cause of most disease and aging. This results in a biochemical transition that actually causes the brain to function in a more youthful manner.

- **Melatonin prevents jet lag and promotes sleep.** More than a hundred studies have confirmed the benefits of melatonin in helping you get to sleep and adjust to a new time zone.

DOSAGE INFORMATION FOR SUPPLEMENTING MELATONIN

- **General nutritional replacement.** I recommend taking 1 to 5 mg before sleep, ideally when the room is already dark. Increase your dose every three to four days, until you feel that you are getting the optimal results, but take no more than 5 mg daily. Decrease your dosage if you experience any of the side effects described in the section that follows.

- **Treating insomnia.** For the treatment of insomnia, begin by taking 1 mg before bedtime, and increase your dosage every two to three days to a maximum of 6 mg. When you try to sleep, make sure your room is quiet and dark, or use eyeshades and earplugs or noise-canceling headphones.

- **Preventing jet lag.** For the treatment of jet lag, begin with the maximum dose that you have tolerated in the past. If you've never taken melatonin, start with 2 mg. When you try to sleep, make sure your room is quiet and dark, or use eyeshades and earplugs or noise-canceling headphones.

- **Getting back to sleep.** Melatonin helps you fall asleep and increases the quality and depth of your sleep, but it does not help you *stay* asleep. If you take melatonin for insomnia and jet lag, and you awake in the middle of the night, do not turn on the lights. In order to fall asleep again, take half the dosage you used to get to sleep.

- **Treating migraine, depression, anxiety, and headache that affect sleep.** For the treatment of these conditions, I recommend supplementing .5 mg or less, increased every three to four days, with your maximum no more than 6 mg. Your dose should be taken before sleep, when your room is already dark. Increase the dose every three to four days. This dosage is also appropriate for using melatonin to improve fertility.

- **Using melatonin to treat cancer and degenerative diseases that can affect sleep.** For the treatment of these conditions, I recommend supplementing 10 to 20 mg daily. In my practice I recommend this supraphysiological dose to patients with unresponsive depression, unresponsive migraine, and tinnitus.

- **Using melatonin with arginine.** Women who take arginine to improve sleep, blood flow to sexual organs, or cardiovascular protection should add melatonin to their arginine treatment in order to balance arginine's production of nitric oxide (NO), a healthy by-product that may also function as a free radical if unchecked. If you supplement arginine, melatonin should be added irrespective of whether you sleep well.

LOW-DOSE SIDE EFFECTS OF MELATONIN

- **Waking with a hangover, or feeling groggy and still sleepy.** Cut down your dose by 1 mg.

- **Waking in the middle of the night, feeling wired.** Melatonin converts thyroid T4 into T3, which causes the body to feel highly wakeful, or "wired." If this occurs, cut your dose to the last amount you took without experiencing this side effect.

- **Nightmares or vivid, intense dreams.** Deep, intense dreaming indicates that you are in the deepest stage of sleep, which is a good thing. If you find that your dreams are *too* intense, simply cut your dosage by 1 mg.

- **Unexpected or opposite-from-expected response.** If you take melatonin to reduce a condition, such as migraine or insomnia, and you find that you experience another migraine or another bout of insomnia, you may be experiencing a paradoxical response that requires you to alter your dose. If you have just started taking melatonin, stop taking it for three to four days and begin taking it again at half the previous dose. If the unusual side effect occurred when you increased your dose, simply reduce your dosage to the level you enjoyed before.

> **Not feeling anything?** Today's lifestyle is defined by immediate gratification. We are accustomed to taking a pill and immediately feeling its power. Unlike conventional medications, natural supplements sometimes require us to be a bit more patient. For example, one of the mech-

anisms by which melatonin helps us get to sleep is a decrease in anxiety and cortisol levels at night. However, enjoying this benefit requires taking melatonin for a number of weeks before we feel a change. If you have built up your dose and are at or near your maximum, but have yet to feel a side effect or a benefit, give melatonin a few weeks before you give up and abandon your daily dosage.

Never worked for you before? Frequently I hear patients say that they have tried melatonin in the past and it didn't work for them, or it resulted in unwanted side effects. Because I am such a strong believer in the overall value of melatonin, I always recommend that they give it another try. The quality of melatonin, dose per capsule, and treatment conditions vary widely. For my own patients, I recommend they start their treatment again with a form of melatonin that I know and have experience with, on the lowest dosage, and following the environmental guidelines described above.

HIGH-DOSE SIDE EFFECTS OF MELATONIN

When I recommend melatonin in supraphysiological doses of 10 to 20 mg, I suggest that patients begin taking 10 mg and increase the dosage to 20 mg a few days later. It is unusual to experience low-dose side effects such as middle-of-the-night awakening or bad dreams when taking high doses of melatonin. Any low-dose side effects with 10 mg often resolve when you double your dose to 20 mg, because high doses of melatonin may bypass the area of the brain that controls sleep.

ACTIVITY MAINTENANCE TO PROMOTE SLEEP

- **Exercise.** Women who exercise regularly also enjoy better quality sleep than those who do not exercise. Physical activity in the evening a few hours before you intend to sleep can be especially useful for calming a racing mind.

- **Relaxing activities.** If you find that your mind races and you cannot fall asleep, but the idea of exercise feels too rigorous before bedtime, consider the opposite extreme—yoga, stretching, Pilates, and meditation may also help you relax enough to quiet your mind and fall asleep.

- **How long does it take to recover from insomnia?** Longer than you think. If you haven't slept well in a long time, and the recommendations found here help, you are likely to find that while you are thankful to be sleeping, you do not feel as perky when you first wake up in the morning. Give yourself some time. It will take your brain a while to catch up on the sleep it requires to feel well rested. You may feel groggy at first, but your brain will adjust once it has had a chance to fully repair and eventually you will feel "perky" again.

 Lisa's Story

Lisa, thirty-five, a young woman who used birth control pills and felt that she was in general good health, visited me at my office and explained that she had not slept well in six months. Her inability to sleep seemed to be getting worse, and had begun to affect her lifestyle. Initially, she was able to successfully treat her insomnia with over-the-counter sleep medication, but even with this help, Lisa was not able to sleep deeply, never dreamt, and generally woke up feeling groggy. After a while these medications stopped working.

My assessment of Lisa's challenge was very simple—she wasn't sleeping because she was on birth control pills. Like any other chemicalized medications, birth control pills contain medications that are not identical to the hormones found in a woman's body. Because Lisa was on the pill, her body was not producing the amount of estrogen that women require in order to sleep well.

Why is this? The chemicals in birth control pills shut down the hormone production of your ovaries, so that you are entirely reliant on the hormones provided by the pills. Today, the chemicalized form of estrogen used in birth control pills is very low. This low dose may be enough to prevent conception, but it is often not sufficient to allow women to sleep. Progesterone is another key hormone that helps women sleep. Unfortunately, bioidentical progesterone is not used in birth control pills, neither is it produced by the ovaries when the pill is taken. On the other hand, not only does the chemicalized progestin or progestogen found in the pill not promote sleep, but it can cause agitation that prevents sleep altogether.

It was obvious to me that Lisa needed to find another means of birth control. It wasn't that the pill was preventing her from sleeping *every* night—Lisa was able to get some relatively nonrestful sleep in the first three weeks of the birth control pill cycle, because her pills contain *some* chemicalized estrogen. But in her placebo week, when Lisa received no chemicalized estrogen from her pill, because her own ovarian hormone production was shut down, Lisa found that she could not sleep at all.

When I spoke to her about my conclusion, Lisa explained that she did not feel comfortable getting off the pill, so I suggested she do the following:

- Supplement bioidentical estrogen in cream form during her birth control pill's placebo week. See Chapter 4 for more information on how to use bioidentical estrogen cream.
- Supplement bioidentical progesterone in sublingual drop form all month long. Many of the properties of bioidentical progesterone are blocked by the mere presence of the chemicalized progesterone replacements found in the pill. Lisa's supplement of progesterone drops will allow her to normally produce GABA and sleep well during the whole month.

Following this protocol, Lisa returned to her pre-pill sleep pattern and sleep quality. I would have been happier if Lisa had agreed to stop taking the pill, but felt satisfied that her modified program allowed her to resolve her sleep disorder without the use of habit-forming sleep medications.

15 • Memory

QUICK QUIZ

Answer the following questions to find out if you greatly need to improve your memory:

Are you forgetful?

Do friends and coworkers report that you are repeating questions?

Do you find that you forget your keys, the bag you meant to take out the door with you, the reason you called friends on the phone?

Do you walk into a room and realize that you don't know why you chose to enter?

Do you find that you have a familiar word in mind that you cannot articulate or pronounce?

Do you accidentally use a word that means the opposite of what you were trying to express?

Have you recently made grammatical mistakes or changes from past to present tense in midsentence?

If you are bilingual, do you find that you begin your sentence in one language, and without realizing it, switch to your other language in order to complete the thought?

Or do you find yourself starting a sentence and forgetting what you meant to say midway through?

Do you have a hard time recalling what you did yesterday?

Do you forget the names of known people, elected officials, popular celebrities?

Do you fail to recognize people you know when you encounter them in an unfamiliar context?

Do you find that you *must* write things down in order to remember to do them? Do you put keys in the same place in order to avoid losing them? Do you find you have to come up with similar systems in order to avoid constantly losing and forgetting things?

Do you miss appointments or forget birthdays?

Do you find that you are more forgetful when you experience stress? When you experience insomnia?

If you relate to the scenarios described above, you may be experiencing some degree of memory loss.

MEMORY BASICS

Memory is everything. You can strive to be the healthiest woman in the world, but without a functioning memory, your overall ability to function is limited, at best.

Despite this, most of us are slowly losing our memories. Some women begin losing their ability to remember at a relatively young age, while others feel a slow decline in their cognitive function over ten or more years. For women who have always enjoyed a great, sharp memory, the loss of any ability to recall details is a big loss; for others who had a poor memory to begin with, losing any memory function may not seem like much, but is nonetheless problematic in their day-to-day life.

Most books devoted to the subject of memory loss focus on end-stage loss in Alzheimer's disease and vascular dementia, in which your brain ceases to function due to lack of oxygen because of a stroke or some other event. In fact, most of the effort in medicine seems to be focused on this group. I have a tremendous amount of compassion for men and women living with Alzheimer's and similar diseases, but this stage of loss is not the focus of this chapter. My aim is to address the *initial* phases of memory loss experienced not only by every Alzheimer's patient, but also by millions of healthy adults every day. Most women who experience this often speak to their physicians about their change of mental function and receive only the following advice:

"Don't worry, you're just stressed."
"You're just working too much."
"You need a vacation."
"Don't take it too seriously. You're over forty, it's normal."
"Everybody goes through this."
"There's nothing you can do."

If this describes you, *you* are the focus of this chapter. In the pages that follow, you will find tools to arrest the decline of your memory, maintain your present level of memory, and restore deficiencies that may allow you to regain some of the memory function you have lost.

There is no magic pill. Our brain and its memory are sensitive and complex. Fully addressing the loss of memory, as in the case of most other "glitches" in this book, requires us to approach all four pillars:

DIET AND NUTRITIONAL SUPPLEMENTS FOR IMPROVING MEMORY

It's possible to write an entire book just on the subject of diet and memory. In this section, I will concentrate on the most important changes you can make to help you *immediately* improve your memory.

1. Reduce your consumption of high-carbohydrate and high-glycemic-index foods. High-carbohydrate, high-glycemic meals don't just put you into a "sugar coma," they actually harm your brain cells. In fact, in addition to being the culprits behind diabetes and insulin resistance, lifestyle complications, and unwanted weight gain, these conditions also happen to be devastating to your brain. Why is this?

Your brain energizes itself with sugar. But just as important as fueling on sugar is the ability to balance sugar levels in your brain. When you develop insulin resistance as a consequence of consuming a high-carbohydrate and high-glycemic diet, your body and brain are unable to properly balance sugar levels. This, in turn, prevents proper brain fueling, but also directly *promotes brain cell destruction.*

Here's how this happens: a protein called PI3 kinase-Akt balances sugar levels in your brain cells by increasing two other proteins: brain-derived neurotrophic factor (BDNF) and NGF (nerve growth factor). The condition of insulin resistance decreases PI3 kinase-Akt and causes your brain sugar levels to become imbalanced, preventing your brain from properly receiving the fuel it requires. In fact, women with Alzheimer's also have decreased levels of PI3 kinase-Akt. At the same time, insulin resistance also increases levels of an enzyme called glycogen synthase kinase 3 (GSK–3), which prevents insulin from communicating with brain receptors charged with feeding your brain, and ultimately causes brain cell loss. Not surprisingly, women with Alzheimer's also have increased levels of GSK–3. As if that weren't bad enough, GSK–3 is also responsible for destroying microtubules and mitochondria, the energy centers of your brain cells. In other words, increasing GSK–3 prevents your brain from properly accessing the sugar energy it needs and also prevents your brain from utilizing any fuel it already has.

As if all this weren't bad enough, insulin resistance also promotes destruction of acetylcholine, a major memory-enhancing neurotransmitter. In other words, if you have diabetes, are prediabetic, or are simply eating a high-carbohydrate, high-glycemic diet, your brain and memory are under significant assault every day.

When the memory and brain function of women with diabetes is tested, the more advanced their condition, the more likely they are to have problems with memory and brain function.

Think just one meal, or one year of these meals doesn't make a difference? Think again. Adults with type 2 diabetes evidence better cognitive performance following *just one* low-glycemic index, low-carbohydrate meal. *Just one.* Now think about how many of these meals you've had during the course of your lifetime.

THE CONNECTION BETWEEN WHAT YOU EAT AND HOW WELL YOU THINK

Did you know a diet that promotes insulin resistance has also been proven to promote amyloids, proteins known to cause Alzheimer's?

Children throughout the world—irrespective of education or socioeconomic condition—are rewarded for good behavior with high-carbohydrate, high-glycemic index food and drink products. By age twelve, a significant percent of the world's children already show evidence of type 2 diabetes. Can you just imagine how their diet affects their cognitive function?

In a study on fruit and vegetable consumption in 3,718 participants, ages sixty-five and older, scientists observed that those who consumed more vegetables experienced a far slower decline in their memory. On the other hand, consumption of fruit did not similarly slow memory decline. Why? Although fruits and vegetables both contain nutrients and antioxidants, fruit has a higher glycemic index, which may explain why it does not similarly benefit memory preservation.

Remember: any time you have a carbo-load or sugar-binge day, you also have a memory-destruction day. I encourage you to think about this the next time someone passes you a piece of party cake and announces: "You only live once!" I agree; you only have one chance to live well.

On the other hand, *every time* you choose a low-carbohydrate, low-glycemic meal, you improve your memory and cognitive function. In addition, the following supplements will directly increase your levels of PI3 kinase-Akt, a protein that promotes memory health:

- **DHEA.** For more information on supplementing this hormone, see Chapter 7.
- **Fish oil** (DHA/EPA). I recommend supplementing 1 to 3 grams, twice daily.
- **Green tea.** I recommend supplementing two to four cups daily or two to four tablets of green tea extract daily.
- **Melatonin.** I recommend supplementing 1 to 6 mg, daily.

Imagine, by simply staying faithful to your diet, supplementing fish oil, eating salmon for dinner, drinking green tea after your meal, or taking melatonin before you go to sleep, you'll be doing a great deal to prevent sugar-induced brain damage and memory loss.

You can also protect your cognitive function by decreasing your levels of GSK–3 with the following supplements:

- **Galantamine** is an herbal remedy that promotes memory and decreases GSK–3. I recommend supplementing 4 to 16 mg daily. For more information, see the discussion of galantamine on page 307.

• **Insulin Balance** is an herbal remedy that decreases incidence of insulin resistance and decreases GSK–3. I recommend supplementing two capsules, twice daily.

2. Choose to eat good fats. For many years, it was not widely accepted that food can have an influence on brain structure and development. I've never believed this; my position has always been that what we eat makes *all* the difference. This is particularly true regarding the types of fats we consume, specifically, whether we consume "good fats" or "bad fats." Good fats are those containing essential fatty acids, also known as omega-3 fats. These fats are found in fish oil. "Bad fats" are sometimes identified as "saturated" and "trans fats." Are you feeding your brain "good fat" or "bad"?

Consider the following:

Research has shown that omega-3 fatty acids provide significant benefits to the brain. On the other hand, diets that are omega-3 deficient can cause structural abnormalities and a decline in cognitive function.

In studies on animals, those found to have the ability to master special memory tasks more quickly were also found to have a higher level of brain-derived neurotrophic factor (BDNF) in the hippocampus section of their brain. Feeding these same animals a "normal" American diet that includes high-fat and high-refined-sugar foods for two months has been shown to decrease their BDNF and their spatial memory function.

In humans, a study of 2,560 adults tested over six years revealed that those who consumed diets including saturated fats and trans fats experienced a decline in cognitive function.

In fact, diets high in saturated fats have been shown to aggravate the outcome of traumatic brain injuries by decreased cognitive function associated with the decrease of BDNF levels. Most disturbingly, studies indicate that it doesn't take long for the consumption of unfavorable fats—saturated and trans fats—to have a negative effect on your cognitive function. In other words, every meal counts, so choose your fats wisely.

3. Consume a nutrient-rich diet or supplement the nutrients you miss. The positive effects of vitamins and minerals on our brain activity have been established. A diet of healthfully prepared whole foods will arm you with many of the nutrients your brain requires; however, nutritional supplements can help you remedy any deficiencies in the event that you are unable to eat all of the foods recommended, or aren't able to eat as well as you'd like all of the time. More specifically:

- **Vitamin B$_1$ (thiamine)** improves cognitive function and is found in sunflower seeds, nuts, oranges, beans and peas, asparagus, cauliflower, and some other cruciferous vegetables. I recommend taking 25 to 100 mg, daily, with food.

- **Vitamins B$_{12}$ and B$_6$** are both directly involved in production of neurotransmitters. The methylated form of B$_{12}$ is the most suitable for improving brain function and is found in clams, beef, trout, salmon, and some fortified vegetarian foods. A deficiency of B$_{12}$ negatively affects brain function at any age. Vitamin B$_6$ should always be taken when supplementing any member of the vitamin B family. I recommend supplementing 1 to 5 mg of B$_{12}$ daily, and 50 to 150 mg of vitamin B$_6$ daily, with food.

- **Vitamin C** is important to neural function, as it is found in high concentration in the nerve endings of the brain. Vitamin C is found in tropical fruits, including guava, papaya, mango, oranges and other citrus, broccoli, cabbage greens, spinach, red and green bell peppers, strawberries, cantaloupe, and tomatoes. I recommend supplementing 1,000 to 5,000 mg daily, with food.

- **Vitamin D$_3$** has the ability to prevent brain cell degeneration and is found in fish oils such as cod, salmon, mackerel, tuna, and sardines, and milk and eggs. Vitamin D is also absorbed by moderate, unprotected sun exposure. I recommend supplementing 1,000 to 5,000 i.u., daily, with food.

- **Vitamin E** contains a component called alpha-tocopherol, which protects the membranes of your nervous system. Vitamin E is found in sunflower seeds, dry roasted almonds, olives, papaya, blueberries, and greens such as Swiss chard, mustard, turnip, and collard greens. I recommend supplementing 400 i.u. daily, with food.

- **Vitamin K** plays an important role in nerve tissue biochemistry. Significant levels of this vitamin are found in leafy greens and cruciferous vegetables, soybeans, and beef. Taking Vitamin K requires you to consult with a nutrition-oriented physician.

- **Lipoic acid,** particularly the R-lipoic acid form, provides you with core brain function protection, which can repair hippocampal memory deficiency and revive the energy centers of your brain cells—both directly combating the destructive effects of GSK–3. Lipoic acid is found in red meat, spinach, and broccoli. I recommend supplementing 50 to 150 mg daily, with food.

- And finally, while it may sound boring, the **multivitamin** that you take every day really does ensure that every brain function that relies on those nutrients indeed gets what it needs. If you skip a day, do so knowing that the complex machine that is your brain will be missing the fuel it relies on. See Chapter 1 for information on what nutrients your multivitamin should contain.

4. Consume minerals in proper balance. While many minerals provide elements required by your body, they must always be consumed in moderation. For example, just as salt is necessary for human survival, too much can cause high blood pressure and other complications. The same holds for other members of the mineral family, specifically:

- **Iron** is necessary for oxygenation and energy production in your brain. Low levels of iron translate into lower energy production and may even cause attention deficit disorder and hyperactivity. On the other hand, too-high levels of iron increase the production of free radicals and may even increase your risk of Alzheimer's.

- **Magnesium** feeds the "electricity" that runs your brain—it's essential for proper synaptic transmission, and brain, enzymatic, and brain cell activity. When magnesium is given to people before open-heart surgery, it decreases the memory loss that is a common side effect of this intense procedure. And even though this mineral is generally protective of overall brain function, overconsumption of magnesium can make you feel sleepy and temporarily diminish your sharp cognitive function.

- **Zinc** is generally helpful to cognitive function. In a study where 15 to 30 mg were given to 387 healthy adults for three months, patients experienced a significant improvement in their spatial working memory and visual memory.

   5. Avoid heavy metals. Heavy metals such as lead, mercury, thallium, and cadmium function as pro-oxidants, meaning they promote the production of the free radicals that lead to inflammation and disease. While a larger discussion of the established harm caused to your brain by exposure to heavy metals is beyond the scope of this book, most simply put: excess heavy metals have no place in your body or your brain and should be avoided in foods and in your immediate surroundings. More specifically, be aware of the type of fish you consume. Canned fish, and other canned foods, contain high levels of heavy metals. Some fresh-caught fish can also contain high levels of mercury. In addition to educating yourself about these foods, make an effort to vary the foods you eat to decrease your chances of consuming these harmful elements.

6. Consume enough protein. A diet rich in protein will supply your brain with the necessary amino acids required to produce neural receptors and protect your brain from toxicity.

The dietary and nutritional supplements outlined here are more than just suggestions, they're the essential requirements for securing your brain function for the long term. The better you eat, the better you'll feel, and the more clearly you'll think. Do you feel fine despite not following these dietary guidelines? You may not feel this way for much longer. Remember, in our relative youth, our bodies and brains are able to sustain a great deal of abuse before the consequences of the damage we've caused are perceivable. But irrespective of whether you notice the changes in your bio- and neural-chemistry, your brain is sustaining nutritional assaults on a daily and hourly basis, and will begin to perceptively decrease brain function *at some point.* I encourage you to take steps today to protect your brain *before* you feel the effects of poor nutrition, as it is much easier to prevent brain function deterioration than to reverse it.

TESTING TO DETERMINE WHETHER YOUR DIET IS LACKING IN NUTRIENTS

When a patient comes into my office and complains of diminished memory, or if my conversation with a patient regarding her diet causes me to be concerned about future mental function, I run a few tests to determine if her diet is providing her with the nutrients she needs, and whether she is eating foods that her body and brain would prefer that she avoid. Do you feel this patient may be you? Consider the following:

1. Is your diet providing you with sufficient vitamin nutrients? By running a blood test that measures the free-radical load in your body, you and your physician will be able to see what nutrients your body has at its disposal to protect against free-radical assault, in addition to actually measuring your level of most vitamins, minerals, amino acids, and antioxidants.

This series of tests is available through nutrition-oriented physicians and other health-care practitioners.

WHAT IS "NORMAL"?

Unfortunately, there are no normal people for science to recruit as test subjects who have not been exposed to poor diet and compromised water and air quality. Doctors establish "normal" based on the population available to them—in many cases made up of the people who frequent hospitals—the sick and the elderly. For this reason, when I look at blood test results, I prefer patients to be on the highest side of "normal" in order for them to benefit from the nutrients or hormones I am testing for.

But what if you eat well? Despite the fact that my practice has a high proportion of super-health-conscious women, it's rare that I see a patient who has optimum levels of antioxidants, trace elements, and vitamins. When I meet a woman who lives a healthy lifestyle and still lacks these essential nutrients, I always consider that she may not be eating enough— or even supplementing enough—of the nutrients her body and brain are craving. In some cases, my patient may be eating well, but even the healthful foods she puts into her body may not be providing her with all of the nutrients she requires, because the foods themselves are exposed to pollutants and poor "diet." For this reason, we must always consider the end result of what our bodies require, not what others have determined is "normal."

---

2. Is your body showing signs of prediabetes or insulin resistance?
In my office, I use a blood test that measures my patients' fasting insulin, hemoglobin A1c, glucose levels, and the ratio between her triglycerides and HDL (high-density lipoproteins, or "good cholesterol"). This test is available through nutrition-oriented physicians and other health-care practitioners.

3. What is your daily consumption of minerals and heavy metals?
Test to determine whether your mineral balance is ideal and your exposure
to heavy metals is low. The treatment of heavy metal poisoning is beyond
the scope of this book; however, I advise my patients to adjust mineral intake according to test results and make a determination about removing,
or chelating, heavy metals from her body if the patient's complaint of
memory loss exceeds what is appropriate for her age. The form of heavy
metal chelation I use is oral kelation that also includes iodine. This test is
available through nutrition-oriented physicians and other health-care
practitioners.

ADDITIONAL NUTRITIONAL SUPPLEMENTS
FOR IMPROVING MEMORY

As discussed, the ideal way to consume the nutrients required by your
brain is to eat a diet rich in vitamins, minerals, and essential oils, and low
in harmful fats, heavy metals, and high-glycemic index foods. Unfortunately, due to the quality of the food available and the way we eat, it is difficult for most of us to get all that we need to properly fuel our brains. If a
patient who seeks to improve her memory is unable to easily meet her nutritional goals by what she eats, I recommend she incorporate nutritional
supplements into her daily consumption to boost the specific vitamins and
minerals described in the sections above.

In addition, the following supplements can provide specific memory
support:

- **Phosphatidylserine.** This nutrient is a phospholipid, or fat, found in
  the inner leaflet of the brain cell membrane, and plays an important
  role in maintaining the proper function of brain cell membranes.
  Phosphatidylserine increases acetylcholine and serotonin, and has
  been shown to significantly improve memory within just six weeks
  of use.

Look for phosphatidylserine derived from soy lecithin. I recommend supplementing 200 to 400 mg, daily, with food. In my clinical experience, I have found this supplement to provide memory support and also elevate mood. For patients who have trouble relaxing before bedtime, I recommend supplementing a higher dose at night, as phosphatidylserine may decrease cortisol levels.

- **Acetyl-l-carnitine.** This is a component of mitochondrial membrane, or layers surrounding the energy center of each cell, which help to maintain the energy produced by cells. Acetyl-l-carnitine can also decrease the free-radical oxidative stress associated with aging, and has been shown to improve spatial memory, and overall cognitive performance in geriatric adults.

I recommend supplementing 1,000 to 2,000 mg, daily, taken with food. In my clinical experience, taking a larger portion of your daily dose in the morning is advisable, as acetyl-l-carnitine can energize you.

- **Ginkgo biloba leaf extract.** If an aging brain could ask a genie to provide whatever is required to improve brain function, she will blink and provide ginkgo. This plant extract improves memory by suppressing and even reversing the production of amyloid beta (Aβ or A-beta), a dominant factor in Alzheimer's. Ginkgo also protects your brain cells from the destructive effects of N-methyl-D-aspartic acid (NMDA), and when given to patients before open heart surgery, ginkgo increases brain oxygen supply, promotes antioxidant production, and inhibits the production of free radicals. Ginkgo has been shown to prevent age-related memory loss, and in tests on patients with mild to moderate Alzheimer's, a relatively low dose of 160 mg of ginkgo increased the test group's cognitive performance better than a similar group that was given the Aricept (donepezil), one of the most popular pharmaceuticals used to treat the disease. For purposes of improving mild memory loss, I recommend supplementing 120 mg twice or three times daily, with food. In cases of more severe memory loss, or for Alzheimer's patients, I recommend 240 mg, twice or three times daily, with food. Side effects associated with ginkgo include mild gastrointestinal discomfort, headache, and dizziness. These unwanted effects may be controlled by reducing your dose. Because ginkgo is a blood thinner, it must be stopped before undergoing any surgical procedure.

- **Huperzine A.** This nutrient is derived from a Chinese plant historically used to treat fever and blood ailments. Today, huperzine A is recognized as a supplement that prevents brain cell degeneration associated with Alzheimer's and other neuron-degenerative diseases. In addition to other protective mechanisms, huperzine A acts as an acetylcholinesterase inhibitor, preventing the breakdown of acetylcholine, a neurotransmitter imperative for proper cognitive function. Huperzine A has been shown to improve memory in adults who suffer from mild memory loss, and may provide greater benefits than pharmaceutical medications like Aricept (donepezil), used to treat Alzheimer's, because of its ability to cross the blood-brain barrier. Studies recommend supplementing 100 to 300 mg, three times daily, with food. If you experience nausea and muscle tension associated with overproduction of acetylcholine, simply reduce your dose to eliminate these side effects.

- **Vinpocetine.** This herbal remedy is commonly used to treat memory loss associated with cerebrovascular and cognitive diseases, in part because it specifically protects the brain from cell destruction.

In my clinical experience with vinpocetine over the last ten years, I have found it to be mildly effective at improving memory. For this reason, I don't begin treatment with this remedy, but I do add it to larger treatment programs. I recommend supplementing 10 to 20 mg daily, with food.

I have found that many of my patients are less likely to continue a program that requires them to take too many pills in any given day, so I recommend a

product called Memory Support that combines acetyl-L-carnitine, phos-
phatidylserine, ginkgo biloba leaf extract, vinpocetine, and huperzine A. I rec-
ommend two pills, taken twice daily.

- **Galantamine.** This herbal formula is derived from flower bulbs and is
  widely marketed as Razadyne, Razadyne ER, Reminyl, and Nivalin.
  Like huperzine A, galantamine functions as an acetylcholinesterase *in-*
  hibitor, preventing the breakdown of acetylcholine, a neurotransmitter
  imperative for proper cognitive function, and is often found to be more
  effective at improving memory than a number of pharmaceuticals currently used to treat Alzheimer's. In fact, caregivers of patients with
  Alzheimer's report that it is easier for them to communicate with and
  care for patients who supplement galantamine, as compared to patients
  on Aricept. Galantamine is also widely used as a remedy for mild memory loss, yielding consistently good results.

  In my clinical experience I have also seen great results. I recommend
  supplementing 4 to 16 mg, daily, taken with food. Begin with 4 mg
  and increase your dose every few weeks. Because galantamine increases
  your supply of acetylcholine, taking too much may cause nausea. Simply reduce your dosage by 4 mg. Most women who supplement other
  memory-support nutrients may never require more than 8 mg, although women who take only galantamine may find that they benefit
  from supplementing up to 16 mg daily.

ADDITIONAL NUTRITIONAL SUPPLEMENTS TO ENHANCE MEMORY

Although they may have entered the mainstream consciousness relatively
recently, the following so-called smart drugs have been found to safely
boost memory and cognitive ability for decades. Many are still used

regularly today. If you would like to try one or more of these smart drugs, I recommend choosing one or two and beginning with those. If one doesn't work for you, another one may. After all, each of us is unique and will not respond in the exact way our friend does. If you experience any side effects or discomforts, simply reduce your dose, and if that is not helpful, simply determine that the smart drug in question is not for you.

- **Hydergine (ergoloid mesylates).** This fungus extract, which has been used to promote memory for more than twenty years, is also marketed under the names Gerimal, Niloric, and Redizork. Studies on very low-dose treatment have shown hydergine to be helpful at improving memory loss, but less so on patients who have already been diagnosed with Alzheimer's. Because hydergine is a MAO inhibitor, it improves the function of neurotransmitters serotonin and dopamine, both destroyed by MAO.

  In my fifteen-year clinical experience with hydergine, I find that it can be helpful in the early stages of memory loss. I recommend supplementing 2.5 to 10 mg, daily, with food, beginning with the lowest dose and increasing gradually. If you experience mild nausea, mild headache, or gastrointestinal symptoms, simply reduce your dosage.

- **Aniracetam and piracetam.** These smart drugs are both derivatives of pyroglutamic acid, an amino acid found in human foods, and have been used to improve memory for more than twenty years. Important for the function of the brain, aniracetam improves memory by increasing your supply of PI3 kinase-Akt, the protein that balances sugar levels and feeds your brain cells. Aniracetam also increases dopamine and serotonin levels, as well as your ability to learn, improves depression, reduces anxiety, and improves sleep. Piracetam has been shown to improve learning and memory in healthy adults. In more extreme cases, aniracetam and piracetam have also been shown to improve memory loss after electroshock therapy, barbiturate intoxication, and even in cases of mild to moderate degrees of amnesia.

I recommend supplementing 750 to 1,500 mg of aniracetam over twenty-four hours and 2,400 to 4,800 mg of piracetam over twenty-four hours. In my clinical experience, side effects are extremely rare. Patients with learning disabilities find it helpful to combine piracetam and hydergine in gel form and apply it twice daily, in the morning and at night.

- **Centrophenoxine (meclofenoxate** or **Lucidril).** This combination of DMAE, a naturally occurring substance found in the human brain, and pCPA, a plant growth hormone, has been available for nearly thirty years. Centrophenoxine improves memory by reducing a residue or pigmentation called lipofuscin that accumulates on your brain cells and decreases their ability to function efficiently. Centrophenoxine also reverses aluminum toxicity associated with Alzheimer's.

  In my fifteen-year clinical experience, I recommend supplementing 500 mg, twice daily, taken with food, although the more brain-support nutrients you take, the less centrophenoxine you'll require.

HORMONAL BALANCE FOR IMPROVING MEMORY

Imagine that your hormones act as an essential component of the engine that "runs" your memory. For this reason, any impairment or less than optimal function of your hormone system negatively affects your ability to enjoy full cognitive function. For example, estrogen is a major component of women's memory engine. Many women notice a significant difference in cognitive ability in the few days leading up to and during their menstrual cycle, when estrogen is low and falling, as compared to the twelfth day of their cycle, when estrogen is high and rising. Does this sound familiar? If so, read on for more about how estrogen affects memory. Other hormones that work intimately with memory include:

- **Thyroid.** If you think that thyroid only affects your energy and ability to lose weight, think again. Thyroid deficiency is always associated with memory disturbance. Studies indicate that even women at the lower end of the normal thyroid production range have significantly more cognitive impairment. In these cases, being in the normal range is irrelevant—the women are deficient because the level they produce is not enough for their bodies. In this way, many women with thyroid deficiencies go undiagnosed. But regardless, the deficiency is very real; in some women with suboptimal thyroid levels, you can see a change in the way the brain looks by MRI and CT scan imaging. The good news is that addressing this memory loss is fairly quick: simply addressing your thyroid deficiency for three months provides a noteworthy improvement to many aspects of cognitive function and verbal memory retrieval. Supplementing natural thyroid should be done with the help of a nutrition-oriented physician who has experience in working with *natural* thyroid supplements.

- **Melatonin.** In Chapter 14, I discussed melatonin's role as a powerful antioxidant, guarding your brain from the destructive effects of free radicals, restoring your brain's hormonal function, and acting as an antidepressant and sleep aid that also helps control cortisol levels at night. In addition, melatonin inhibits the generation of beta-amyloid and tau hyperphosphorylation, two serious markers that define Alzheimer's. In other words, maintaining proper levels of melatonin is essential to your brain's health.

For patients with mild memory loss, I recommend supplementing .5 to 10 mg, daily, with food. For those with more significant memory loss, I recommend 10 to 20 mg, daily, with food. See Chapter 14 for more specific information on beginning treatment with melatonin.

- **DHEA and testosterone.** Both of these androgen hormones are helpful in improving memory, as follows:

  - DHEA increases PI3 kinase-Akt, the protein that helps balance brain sugar levels and protects the brain from the devastating effects of a high-glycemic-index diet.
  - DHEA suppresses high cortisol levels.
  - DHEA converts to estrogen, the hormone that is most supportive to memory, as you will read about below.
  - DHEA acts as an antidepressant, and in doing so improves memory.
  - DHEA and testosterone uniquely protect against Alzheimer's by minimizing the devastating affects of a lipoprotein called apolipoprotein E4, present in 20 percent of the general population, but present in the majority of Alzheimer's patients. For this reason, women with a family history of Alzheimer's should always check for the presence of this lipoprotein.
  - Like DHEA, testosterone can also directly improve memory. In studies, supplementing low-dose testosterone in adults—even healthy young women—significantly improved these women's visual and spatial memory.

Taking DHEA or testosterone for any reason requires individualized dosing information, available in Chapters 7 and 9.

- **Progesterone.** The bioidentical form of progesterone serves as a wonderful aid that improves memory by calming you, improving your sleep, and providing significant general cognitive protection by increasing BDNF and decreasing glutamate toxicity. In the growing research field on brain trauma, progesterone has been shown to prevent damage caused by trauma and to enhance the rate and extent of recovery. Demand the best care available to you, and if that includes improving your memory with bioidentical progesterone, I encourage you not to accept the response "You don't need it."

For more information about how bioidentical progesterone can improve your memory, and why chemicalized progesterone alternatives cannot, see the discussion of memory in Chapter 5.

- **Estrogen.** Estrogen promotes memory function in a number of ways:

  - As a MAO inhibitor, estrogen improves serotonin and norepinephrine levels, reducing depression and anxiety and allowing you to feel more clearheaded.
  - Estrogen increases brain growth factor, which improves the rate of neuronal survival.
  - Estrogen maintains the connection between the brain cells.
  - Estrogen increases blood flow to the brain.
  - Estrogen increases the production of dopamine.
  - Estrogen treatment causes the area of the brain responsible for higher mental function to become highly active.

Supplementing estrogen for any reason requires individualized dosing information, available in the discussion of memory in Chapter 4.

- **Pregnenolone.** This hormone positively affects memory in a number of ways: it stimulates cell production in the hippocampus area of the brain, and also protects brain cells in the hippocampus, the thinking area of the brain, from the destructive effects of glutamate and amyloid beta protein toxicity, the genesis of Alzheimer's.

Supplementing pregnenolone for any reason requires individualized dosing information, available in the discussion on memory in Chapter 8.

- **Human growth hormone (HGH).** HGH works as an incredible brain booster. Unfortunately, most of us are deficient in our production of this crucial hormone. Studies on HGH and memory enhancement focus on people with severe HGH deficiency, and therefore call for very high doses of this hormone. In my practice, I am able to treat relatively healthy patients with significantly lower doses, and these patients often find that they are able to concentrate for longer periods of time, retain more information, and enjoy overall superior brain vitality.

  Unfortunately, after estrogen, HGH is the hormone that has received the second-worst reputation. For more information on why HGH is safe, including individual dosing protocols under the care of a physician, see Chapter 6.

ACTIVITY CONSIDERATIONS FOR IMPROVING MEMORY

- **Simple mental exercises.** Studies indicate that older adults who continue to engage their brains even with simple pastimes such as brain teasers and verbal memory training techniques are able to maintain and improve their memory and larger cognitive function. In younger women, these same memory-engaging techniques can also be helpful in correcting memory loss.

  In other words: Use it or lose it. You must make a concerted effort to continue engaging your brain. Open a book of poetry and memorize a few lines. Do a crossword puzzle or solve a Sudoku grid every day. If you come across a word whose meaning you do not know or cannot recall, immediately look it up—the process of teaching or reminding yourself will get you back in the habit of retrieving data. These exercises are a "cardio workout" for your brain.

- **Exercises to improve consolidation.** If you find that you are repeatedly unable to recall a given name, write this name or other information on a card and place it in your wallet or on a page in your planner. Read this name to yourself every day. This technique improves cognitive consolidation, the process that stores information in the area of your brain that allows you to retrieve it at will. Practicing on one name also improves your overall ability to consolidate all information you come in contact with.

- **Social and professional activity.** Staying in touch with others, including a connection to the professional world, even after retirement or a child-rearing-related hiatus, is essential to maintaining memory and larger cognitive function. Retirees are often encouraged to prepare themselves for retirement with a new "job." Expectant mothers should do the same, by setting up a social or professional network they will interact with once they begin their new schedule.

- **Physical activity to improve memory.** Surprisingly, moving the body significantly improves learning, memory, and overall cognitive function. Studies indicate that consistent treadmill running improves the rate of brain cell production in the hippocampus, the thinking center of the brain.

Additionally, exercise improves the levels of other proteins that combat the negative effects of a high-fat diet. In studies on healthy women between the ages of fifty-nine and sixty-eight, participants significantly improved their cognitive performance after only three months of exercise, particularly in the area of face-name association. A combination of "mental training" and aerobic training evidences a greater improvement than either mental or physical training alone. The good news is that anything that benefits a relatively older Natural Superwoman, significantly benefits a younger woman far more readily.

See Chapter 2 for more information on how to moderate exercise without compromising other health goals.

MIND AND MOOD CONSIDERATIONS
FOR IMPROVING MEMORY

In general, our quality of sleep, level of stress, and sense of happiness all have a profound effect on our memory function. Just two weeks of healthy lifestyle programs that improve sleep and include a balanced diet, exercise, relaxation exercises, and mental and cardiovascular exercises have been shown to significantly improve cognitive function. In other words, how you feel in general has everything to do with how your memory performs.

HOW STRESS AFFECTS YOUR MEMORY

If you think being stressed out negatively affects your ability to remember, you're right. The effect of stress on memory is significant and dramatic. Stress is associated with changes in the hippocampal function and structure, which means that it actually changes the function and structure of the area of the brain charged with managing memory and thought. Experiencing stress decreases brain cell production, increasing production of cortisol, the fight-or-flight hormone that encourages you to run, not to stop and think, and decreasing brain-derived neurotrophic factor (BDNF). In fact, in posttraumatic stress disorder, atrophy sets into the white matter of the brain and hippocampal volume is reduced. That's right, it's not your imagination, the size of your brain actually shrinks as a consequence of stress.

Additionally, psychological stress has been shown to impair working memory and decrease ability to retrieve stored information, preventing you from remembering names, faces, and places. And, in general, daily stress is associated with decreased mental performance in healthy adults. In studies, the more interpersonal stress adults experience, the greater their rate of memory failure on a day-to-day basis.

My aim is not to scare you into feeling bad about what memory capacity you may have lost the last time you experienced stress. I'm not suggesting that you leave your family for a life of bliss at a meditation retreat. That's not realistic for me, and probably not for you. My goal is to make you aware of the consequences of putting pressure on your mind and body, and to arm you with tools to combat the real pressures that most of us must confront on a daily basis. In doing so, you can recapture much of the function you enjoyed before.

What can you do to recover memory loss?

Studies indicate that yoga, prayer, tai chi, and meditation are all mind and mood activities that assist the brain in healing. And while few Natural Superwomen have the luxury of practicing tai chi or yoga while in a meeting or shuttling around a young family, the principles of breath regulation outlined in Chapter 11 go a long way toward connecting you with the healing properties of these activities, and can be done nearly anytime or anywhere.

Of course, the nature of the strong superachiever is that she often wants what she cannot have, or what is not practical, and this instinct can cause stress all on its own. I encourage you to keep in mind that the power to regulate your breath is something that you can call on and employ at any time to help achieve your other goals. You may be annoyed that I keep reminding you to breathe, over and over again, but in my clinical practice I find that's the case with my busiest, most competent, and smartest patients. Why is this? I believe that the instinctive response to stress is to run, not to relax and breathe thoughtfully. So even if you know that breathing is good for you, the moment of stress may blind you to this. If you feel that your cognitive function has diminished since the onset of a period of greater stress in your lifestyle, review Chapter 11.

HOW LACK OF SLEEP AFFECTS YOUR MEMORY

Studies clearly establish that sleep deprivation is a chronic stress inducer that also contributes to diminished cognitive function. I'm sure you're nodding as you read this—you already know that your mind is more likely to draw a blank if you are sleep deprived. Sleep deprivation impairs spatial memory and also impairs hippocampal function. Sleep apnea, a condition that disrupts sleep and nighttime oxygen intake, is a growing problem among adults and has been associated with memory loss as well. Resolving sleep apnea with the use of a positive airway pressure (PAP) mask restores much of the lost cognitive function associated with this condition.

If you feel that your cognitive function has diminished since the onset of a period of reduced sleep, review Chapter 14.

HOW ABSENCE OF WELL-BEING OR DEPRESSION AFFECTS YOUR MEMORY

There is a well-established association between depression, aging, and a subsequent decline in cognitive function. Very nearly everything about depression is destructive to the brain. When you feel depressed, you tend to sleep less well or not at all; experience more stress; eat a higher-carb diet; exercise less or not at all; and spend time in bed, rather than "exercising" your brain.

As an obstetrician, the twenty-five years of my career that I spent delivering babies and functioning on a sleep-deprived basis should have left me with severely diminished mental function. Despite all this, my passion for physical activity, healthy diet, hormone balance, focus on stress reduction techniques, and a great wife have somehow managed to salvage some of my brain cells. In other words, each of us has within us the tools to correct our impairments. Quick fixes are not the answer. I encourage you to examine your lifestyle choices to determine which decisions may be causing your low mood. Just as your reason for sleeplessness is not likely to be an Ambien deficiency, and your depressed condition or feelings of stress are probably not due to a Prozac or Xanax deficiency, respectively, your memory loss is not going to be explained by an Aricept deficiency. A few of us may require these aids for a short- or longer-term period, but remember, these are tools, not solutions. Your real solution lies within *you*.

If you feel that your cognitive function has diminished since the onset of a period of a reduced sense of well-being or depression, review Chapter 12.

Finally, in a UCLA study on how short-term lifestyle changes affect memory, healthy women between the ages of thirty-five and sixty-nine with mild complaints of memory dysfunction were asked to incorporate a brain-healthy eating plan, relaxation exercises, cardiovascular conditioning, and verbal memory training techniques. Researchers found that after just two weeks of addressing the four pillars, these women were able to significantly improve their cognitive function. The bottom line is that small four-pillars changes can make a big difference to you—in some cases in just a few weeks. Who wouldn't try that?

Part Four

Living
Disease-Free
as a Natural
Superwoman

Throughout this book I encourage you to live like a Natural Super-woman by addressing the conditions and discomforts that, while not life-threatening, slow you down and prevent you from operating at your fullest, living at your most happy, and enjoying the people and activities you love.

Natural Superwoman living also incorporates simple, daily good habits that allow you to avoid larger diseases, which may not have noticeable symptoms but are nonetheless threatening to your ability to enjoy life. In this part of the book, I will discuss the small changes you can make in order to proactively protect against and confront "the big O"—osteoporosis—and "the big C"—breast cancer.

16 • Your Bone Health and How to Fight Against Osteoporosis

WHAT CAUSES OSTEOPOROSIS?

According to the National Institutes of Health, osteoporosis is a major public health threat for 28 million Americans, 80 percent of whom are women. Women lose bone for the following reasons:

- Poor diet and lack of vitamins and minerals.
- Inflammation.
- Vitamin D deficiency. In avoiding sun exposure to minimize risk of skin cancer, many women experience other complications due to vitamin D deficiency.
- Magnesium deficiency.
- Lack of exercise.
- Deficiency of estrogen, DHEA, HGH, and testosterone.
- Use of very low-dose birth control pills, which decreases the overall level of estrogen available to the women who take these pills.
- Use of Depo-Provera.
- Use of acid-blocking medications, known as proton pump inhibitors (PPI), used to treat ulcers, gastroesophageal reflux disease

(GERD), and other conditions caused by stomach acid. These drugs includ Protonix (pantoprazole), Prilosec (omeprazole), Prevacid (lansoprazole), and Rabeprazole (Aciphex).

- Use of antidepressant medications from the group known as SSRI, including Prozac, Zoloft, and Lexapro.
- Use of aromatase inhibitors, a common treatment for breast cancer.

This seems like a long list, but if you look more closely you'll see that the causes of osteoporosis connect to things that you may do every day—from what you eat, to your choice of birth control, medications, and activity level. You'll also note that whether you choose to optimize your level of estrogen and other hormones plays a role, as well.

CONVENTIONAL OSTEOPOROSIS TREATMENTS

To any woman who watches television, it may seem that the simple solution to osteoporosis can be found in oral medications like Fosamax and Boniva. Sounds easy, right? The truth is these drugs have serious side effects. Among them is a risk for significant damage to your esophagus. For this reason, users are instructed not to lie down within thirty minutes of taking these medications and, if esophageal discomfort does occur, to immediately stop taking the medication and consult with their physicians.

The more serious problem with these medications is a risk of developing jawbone necrosis, where you may develop holes in your jaw, and in extreme cases, *have to have your jaw removed*. It is common for medical experts to downplay the frequency of these extreme side effects, yet jaw damage is one of the most common malpractice suits brought by patients against the manufacturers of these drugs.

In addition, osteoporosis medications have no means of exiting the body after use. Most medications are metabolized by the liver. The osteoporosis medication group either exits the body in your urine, or accumulates in your bones. The longer you use these medications, the more will accumulate in your bones and remain there for decades. The idea of medications accumulating in women's bones is of extreme concern to me. After all, your bones were not designed to house these medications, and, more disturbing, the buildup of these medications may eventually displace women's bone marrow.

Also, while this medication group stops bone loss very effectively, in doing so, it also effectively *decreases the building of new bone by 60 to 90 percent.* Because of this, if you fracture a bone while taking medications in this group, you may experience slow and inefficient healing during the time you are taking these medications. These effects can last up to five years after you stop taking the drugs.

Finally, long-term use of this medication group may lead to arterial plaque instability and cardiovascular events, such as stroke and heart attack.

- **Natural osteoporosis treatments.** In my practice, I do not prescribe osteoporosis medications; instead, I do the following:

  - Review the patient's diet.
  - Test blood for antioxidant–free radical balance.
  - Conduct genomic testing that identifies genetic risk factors for osteoporosis.
  - Check level of magnesium, trace elements, inflammation markers, and all relevant hormones.

For patients who are indeed experiencing bone loss, I recommend a regimen of natural supplements and exercise.

SUPPLEMENTS TO PREVENT
AND TREAT OSTEOPOROSIS

The following natural supplements can help you prevent and treat osteoporosis. Your nutrition-oriented physician can advise you about how many of these should be added to your supplement program:

- **High-quality, low-mercury fish oil (DHA & EPA).** I recommend 2,000 mg, twice daily, with food.

- **Highly-absorbable magnesium**, such as magnesium glycinate. I recommend 200 to 1,000 mg, twice daily, taken with food.

- **High-dose vitamin D$_3$.** I recommend 5,000 mg daily, with food, for six weeks, monitored closely for vitamin D blood levels with the dose readjusted accordingly, followed by 5,000 mg three times *weekly*, with food. Note that supplementing vitamin D$_3$ in menopausal or perimenopausal women may increase calcification, for this reason I always add vitamin K$_2$ to protect against this.

- **High-quality, high-quantity vitamin K$_2$** as a preventative treatment for osteoporosis and arterial calcification. This nutrient removes calcium from the artery and increases it in the bone, and has been used for years in Japan to treat both osteoporosis and cardiovascular disease. Although some vitamin K$_2$ supplements can be inefficient and expensive, the vitamin K$_2$ I use in my office provides high quality, quantity, purity, and efficiency at a relatively low cost. I recommend supplementing 75 to 150 mcg daily, with food. Be sure to look for K$_2$ identified as MK-7 (menaquinone-7), the only natural bioidentical form of K$_2$.

- **Strontium** is an effective bone builder in both the spine and the hips. It also slows bone loss. I recommend 1,000 mg, twice daily with food.

- **Boron** has a mild to moderate effect on bone buildup. I recommend 20 mg, twice daily with food.

ACTIVITIES TO PREVENT AND TREAT OSTEOPOROSIS

- **Weight-bearing exercise**, such as light weightlifting, is encouraged for building bone.

- **Hormones to prevent and treat osteoporosis.** Optimizing your levels of the following bioidentical hormones can help you prevent and treat osteoporosis.

- **Estrogen** and **DHEA** decrease bone loss, while **HGH, testosterone**, and **progesterone** increase bone buildup. See the section for each of these hormones for specific dosing information. Always use these hormones under the care of a physician who has experience in treating osteoporosis with bioidentical hormones.

- **Calcitonin**, a hormone available by prescription from traditional pharmacies under the brand name Miacalcin, is sold as a nasal spray and helps increase buildup of bone in the spine only.

By using a nutritional and bioidentical hormonal approach you can help your existing bone health and repair bone loss. I encourage you to explore these effective alternatives to conventional osteoporosis medications.

17 • Strategies for Proactively Preventing and Treating Breast Cancer

If you watch television or read mainstream newspapers, chances are you believe that, irrespective of your genetic predisposition, breast cancer is coming for you—it's just a matter of time. Studies indicate that women's fears of how likely they are to develop breast cancer far exceed reality. In today's antiestrogen climate, most women *and their physicians* believe that the culprit behind breast cancer is women's production of estrogen.

The reason breast cancer appears at the end of this long section on the safety of bioidentical hormones is that I want to bring together all the information in these chapters to assure you that when properly balanced, bioidentical hormones do not cause breast cancer and, in fact, can prevent and protect you from this disease.

BREAST CANCER BASICS

Why do women get breast cancer? As it turns out, the risk factors are less mysterious than you might think. In some cases, the causes may be attributed to genetics and events that occurred before your birth, but many times decreasing risk is directly linked to the choices you make every day. In the following section I am not addressing the rare and highly publicized genetic risk factors called *breast cancer 1, early onset* (BRCA1) and *breast cancer 2, early onset* (BRCA2). These genetic predispositions affect relatively few women as compared to other risks, and more importantly, they are well known by the medical community. My aim is to focus on the lesser-known risks that are often overlooked and that affect every woman reading this book. Incidence of breast cancer increases due to the following:

- **Risk factors in utero.** Before you were even born, your risks for developing breast cancer were affected by your mother's environment and choices:

  - **Maternal diet and environmental exposure** during pregnancy *increase* the risk of future adult breast cancer in unborn daughters. A high-fat diet and significant weight gain during pregnancy are two factors.
  - **Alcohol consumption during pregnancy** *increases* the risk of future adult breast cancer in unborn daughters.
  - **Use of diethylstilbestrol (DES)**, a chemicalized estrogen given to women in the United States to decrease the incidence of miscarriage, *increases* the occurrence of breast cancer in their unborn daughters.

  In general, a mother's behavior in pregnancy can have a significant effect on her daughter's risk for developing breast cancer. For more information on a Natural Superwoman–compliant eating program for pregnant women, see my previous book, *How to Make a Pregnant Woman Happy* (Chronicle Books).

- **Adult weight management.** General weight management throughout your life also affects your chances of developing breast cancer. In a study on 87,143 women who were followed for twenty-six years, adult women who gained more than fifty-five pounds since their eighteenth birthdays experienced a significant increase in risk of developing breast cancer. In the same study, women who gained more than twenty-two pounds since entering menopause also experienced an increased risk of developing breast cancer.

• **Food choices.** Although it may not be surprising to you that food choices affect your risk of developing breast cancer, understanding *exactly what* foods and *how much* of them make a difference is eye-opening. For example, "junk food" really matters. Consumption of omega-6, a "bad" fat found in safflower oil, sunflower oil, and corn oil, common in fried and processed foods, significantly increases your risk of developing breast cancer. Similarly, the type of protein you consume directly affects breast cancer risk as well. Studies show eating red meat five or more times a week increases your risk of developing breast cancer by more than 40 percent.

Also, if you eat more than one and a half servings of red meat a day, you increase your risk of developing breast cancer by 97 percent.

The average American family consumes red meat at least once a day. Should the Food and Drug Administration require "black box" warnings on packaging of ground beef? Should burger joints monitor the number of times a week that individuals visit and recommend their chicken sandwich alternative as a public health measure? My point in sharing this statistic is not to scare women away from beef consumption, but to simply highlight that *so many* aspects of our daily diet put women at significant risk of developing breast cancer.

• **Use of oral contraceptives by teenagers.** While adult women have been told to stop taking all estrogen due to studies that evidence an increased risk associated with chemicalized hormones, teenage women have not been educated about the risks associated with their use of chemical hormones. Research shows that young women, ages fifteen to twenty, who use oral contraceptives increase their lifetime breast cancer rate by 15 percent for every year of use. This means a young woman may increase her lifetime breast cancer risk as much as 75 percent by simply taking birth control pills between the ages of fifteen and twenty.

- **Weight management during pregnancy.** As discussed above, the amount of weight and girth you gain during your pregnancy also affects your risk of developing breast cancer. Studies have shown that women who gain more than thirty-eight pounds during pregnancy experience a 48 percent increase in the risk for developing breast cancer. This increased risk is equal to or higher than that for breast cancer associated with studies on use of chemicalized hormones. I wonder how many obstetricians frame their recommendation for maximum weight gain during pregnancy in this context?

  After pregnancy, women whose postpartum (after delivery) waist circumference exceeds 34 inches as a consequence of improper weight management during pregnancy experience a 30 percent increase in their risk of developing breast cancer, as compared with women whose waist circumference is 28 inches.

- **Antibiotic treatment.** The *Journal of the American Medical Association* reports that use of antibiotics for one to fifty days cumulatively throughout your lifetime is associated with a 45 percent increase in your risk of developing breast cancer; using antibiotics cumulatively for 101 to 500 days increases your risk by 68 percent, and 501 to 1,000 cumulative days by 100 percent. This increased breast cancer risk may relate to the proliferation of abnormal bacteria caused by the antibiotics clearing out all gastrointestinal bacteria, including much-needed friendly bacteria.

- **Environmental considerations.** Certain groups of women are naturally more susceptible to environmental pollutants and have an increased risk for developing breast cancer.

- **Stress.** A Danish study on nearly 1,500 women who were followed up for twenty-four years established that those experiencing significant stress doubled their risk of breast cancer.

- **Iodine deficiency.** Multiple studies have demonstrated the association between iodine deficiency and breast disease and cancer. In my practice, when I check iodine levels, I find that nearly 90 percent of my patients are iodine deficient. Your nutrition-oriented physician can design a comprehensive program to address your iodine deficiency.

- **Selective Serotonin Reuptake Inhibitor (SSRI) medications.** Taking SSRI medications, such as Prozac, doubles the incidence of an uncommon yet aggressive type of breast cancer that is estrogen-receptor positive and progesterone-receptor negative.

The Development Time of Cancer

When I ask patients how long they think it takes for initial cell mutation to become a cancerous growth that can be felt by a manual breast exam, most answers are between three months and three years. Cancer actually takes far longer to develop than that: it takes an average of fifteen years from the moment two cells change into cancer cells to the time a cancerous growth measures 1 centimeter, or about $\frac{3}{8}$ inch, when it is able to be felt during a breast exam administered by you or your doctor. It takes an average of ten years for the growth to reach 1 mm, or about $\frac{1}{25}$ inch in size. If you are fortunate and this small breast growth has absorbed calcium, this size is the smallest that can be observed by mammogram. If a woman is diagnosed at age fifty, this woman's breast cancer began developing when she was thirty-five. However, to arrive at the moment when her two healthy cells turn into breast cancer cells required years of multiple biochemical changes. In other words, although a woman may have developed her first breast cancer cell in her midthirties, the process required to arrive at the point where her healthy cells turned into breast cancer cells likely started when she was much younger.

Where Levels of Estrogen Count

Despite fears about the connection between estrogen levels and cancer, nature has been increasing women's estrogen levels in a cancer-free way for all of human history. In pregnancy, estrogen levels rise sky-high, and as a consequence, women's risk of developing breast cancer drops and their rate of survival from breast cancer rises.

The truth is, the amount of estrogen found in your bloodstream is not the concern, but the amount found locally, in your breast tissue. In general, the amount of estrogen found in an adult women's breast tissue is as high as twentyfold of what is found in her bloodstream, irrespective of whether she takes hormones, birth control pills, or is pregnant. Women's breasts simply evidence higher levels of estrogen.

Why are estrogen levels so much higher in breast tissue? It's because of a process called aromatization, where the testosterone found in breast tissue is converted to estrogen. This process is promoted by inflammation, which causes an increase in nuclear factor-kappa beta (NFkB), interleukin-6 and 12, and COX2 (COX-2) activity. Pollutants in diet and the environment increase inflammation, and thus exacerbate the risk of breast cancer.

How Estrogen Metabolizes and How This Relates to Environmental-Sensitivity Breast Cancer

How estrogen metabolizes individually has to do with genetic predisposition, which can also inform susceptibility to breast cancer, and more important, ideal prevention and treatment avenues for your unique individual and genetic risk profile. For more information on diagnosis and treatment, see the "Estrogen Metabolism" section at www.UzziReissMD.com.

PREVENTING AND TREATING BREAST CANCER WITH THE FOUR PILLARS

Diet and Nutrition Pillar

Foods and Food Products to Protect Against Breast Cancer

- **DHA/EPA fish oil.** Perimenopausal women who consume more omega-3 oil (fish oil) and less omega-6 oil (less favorable oil) are 41 percent less likely to develop breast cancer. Simply switching from eating mostly beef to mostly fish will provide you with significantly more breast cancer protection. The results of these studies strongly promote eating more fish and less unfavorable oil. I recommend 2,000 mg, twice daily, with food.

- **Conjugated linoleic acid (CLA).** In lab studies, when CLA was added to a culture of breast cancer cells, it inhibited cell proliferation. I recommend 1,000 mg, twice daily, with food.

- **Flaxseed.** Perimenopausal women who increase the amount of flaxseed in their diet reduce their incidence of breast cancer. Additionally, lignan, a nutrient found in flaxseed, is known to decrease incidence of estrogen-positive progesterone-negative breast cancer, a rare but aggressive form of the disease. Most women find flaxseed tasty and an easy quick addition to salads and smoothies.

- **Whey protein** and whey acid protein, a large component of whey. In studies, this protein inhibits the proliferation of breast cancer. I recommend drinking protein shakes with whey as the protein source or adding whey protein to smoothies.

- **Soy and soy products.** Soy is high in isoflavone genistein, a weak phyto-estrogen that protects against cancer and suppresses the expression of HER-2/neu, an aggressive and hard-to-treat form of this disease.

- **Ginger.** Gingerol, a component of ginger root, inhibits the ability of tumors to become resistant to chemotherapy. For this reason, consuming ginger as a component of your overall chemotherapy program may be helpful for treating tumors that would otherwise be resistant and because ginger has strong antinausea properties. I recommend adding unsweetened ginger to your soups, teas, and other foods.

- **Curcumin, the yellow pigment of the turmeric spice.** This spice component has a strong anti-inflammatory and antitumor effect. I recommend adding this spice to meats and other foods.

- **Green tea.** This popular beverage is currently being investigated as a potential treatment for breast cancer. It is both an anti-inflammatory and COX-2 inhibitor and decreases the aggressive nature of breast cancer cells. Green tea inhibits the destructive effects of an aggressive and hard-to-treat form of breast cancer and suppresses epidermal growth factor receptor (EGFR), which promotes the spread of tumors. Additionally, green tea enhances the efficiency of Taxol (paclitaxel), a chemotherapy drug used in the treatment of breast cancer. I recommend buying decaffeinated green tea and sipping it throughout the day.

- **Grape juice, grape seeds, and red wine.** Grape juice, grape seeds, and red wine extract are all strong aromatase inhibitors. Studies conducted at the City of Hope Cancer Center in Los Angeles established that these compounds' aromatase-inhibiting activity is close to that of other medications used in the treatment of breast cancer, without the toxic effects of those drugs.

  Resveratrol, also found in red wine, is a polyphenolic antioxidant present in grapes, and has potent cancer prevention benefits. It is also a

COX-2 inhibitor and an NFkB inhibitor, and regresses tumor formation at every stage of breast cancer. Researchers studying this component of red wine concluded that resveratrol should be considered as a potent tool in breast cancer treatment. This component of red wine is also considered to be one of the reasons for the "French paradox," an observation that French people—known for drinking one of their national products—eat more fat, smoke, and fail to exercise as much as other populations and nonetheless have relatively low rates of lung cancer, breast cancer, and heart disease.

I recommend drinking one glass (four ounces) of high-quality red wine daily, or supplementing grape seed or red wine extract.

- **Pomegranate.** Various components of pomegranate fruit extract have strong antioxidant and anti-inflammatory properties and decrease NFkB and breast cancer cell proliferation. Extract of this fruit has been proposed as an addition to the treatment of breast cancer. Additionally, pomegranate extract prevents cancer cells from developing new blood vessels that will allow them to spread.

In my practice, I recommend Body Guard as a universal anti-inflammatory for a variety of disease prevention. It is a powder that combines pomegranate, resveratrol, grape seed extract, green tea extract, and curcumin. I find that this combination effectively blocks the avenues used by breast cancer to start, develop, and progress. I suggest that women with active breast cancer take eight to twelve pills twice daily, with food. For women with a family history of breast cancer, or women in remission from breast cancer, I recommend six to eight capsules twice daily, with food, and for general prevention, two to four pills, twice daily, with food.

- **Mushrooms in the *Coprinus comatus*, *Coprinellus* species, and *Flammulina velutipes* species.** All three of these mushroom types promote potent antitumor activity that affects both estrogen receptor positive tumors and estrogen receptor negative tumors. This presents an important remedy option for women with estrogen receptor negative tumors, as these tumors have limited treatment options other than chemotherapy.

- **Mushrooms in the *Ganoderma lucidum* species.** This species of mushrooms inhibits breast cancer by down-regulating NFkB and estrogen receptor, which brings down the amount of estrogen in the breast tissue.

- **Dietary fiber.** In studies of perimenopausal women, consuming more than 30 grams of fiber a day decreased incidence of breast cancer by 50 percent.

NUTRITIONAL SUPPLEMENTS TO PROTECT AGAINST BREAST CANCER

In my practice, I recommend the following supplements for protecting against breast cancer. If you are already taking supplements, I do not recommend that you stop taking those in favor of any one supplement listed below. Simply check what doses of the following are provided by your current supplements and add those that you require or that you require more of. After all, cancer is too big and too complicated. To give yourself the best chance of fighting this devastating disease, you will need to avail yourself of every nutritional tool.

- **DIM (di-indolmethane) and I3C (indole-3-carbinol).** These nutrients, derived from cabbage, increase your level of 2-hydroxy-estrone, an estrogen metabolite that protects against and may even treat breast cancer. Additionally, I3C may markedly reduce epidermal growth factor receptors, which strongly promote the development and spread of breast cancer cells. For information on dosage, see the "Estrogen Metabolism" section at www.UzziReissMD.com.

- **SGS (sulphoraphane glucosinolate).** This extract of cruciferous vegetables such as brussels sprouts and broccoli is a powerful new nutritional tool in the prevention and treatment of breast cancer. For information on dosage, see the "Estrogen Metabolism" section at www.UzziReissMD.com.

- **Quercetin.** This supplement, found in citrus fruit and other foods, helps slow the growth of cancer cells, I recommend eating the white portion of the interior citrus fruit skin, which is rich in quercetin. In supplement form, I recommend 500 mg, twice daily, with food.

- **Selenium.** This supplement decreases the function of the receptor that causes cancer to grow. I recommend checking your selenium level to demonstrate that you are deficient or at the lower end of normal. I always aim to keep breast cancer patients and those with a higher risk of developing the disease on the high end of normal. I suggest taking 100 to 200 mcg, once or twice a day, with food. As a whole food alternative, one organic Brazil nut provides you with 100 mcg of selenium.

- **Vitamin E.** Two forms of vitamin E protect against breast cancer. The first is vitamin E in combination with omega-3 fish oil (DHA/EPA), which restores normal breast cancer cell function. The more cancer cells function and look like noncancerous cells, the less aggressive they are and the more responsive they are to treatment. This may also be a significant preventative of the initiation of the cancer development process. I recommend a supplement that includes the broad range of vitamin E types, alpha, delta, and gamma tocopherol, 400 to 800 mg daily, with food.

Vitamin E tocotrienol is a subgroup of vitamin E that functions as a potent anticancer mechanism in breast precancerous and cancer cells.

This type of vitamin E should be in the treatment program of every breast cancer patient. I recommend a supplement that includes both 90 percent of the delta form and 10 percent of the gamma tocotrienol form extracted from the annatto plant, 100 mg, once or twice a day, with food.

- **Vitamin D$_3$.** This nutrient decreases the growth of breast cancer cells. Our culture is now obsessed with avoiding sun exposure in order to minimize the serious condition of melanoma. However, in doing so, most of us become vitamin D deficient. The deficiency is associated with increased incidence of breast and prostate cancers. For this reason, it is so important to safely supplement vitamin D$_3$. I recommend checking your vitamin D blood level to see whether you are deficient, and then taking steps to bring yourself to the upper level of normal. An inexpensive way to do this is to expose your skin to the sun without sunscreen for a half-hour a day. Plan this time during the hours when the sun is less strong.

- **Coenzyme Q$_{10}$.** In a dramatic report, this supplement was demonstrated to produce complete and partial remission of breast cancer when the patient supplemented 90 to 300 mg daily. Most coenzyme Q$_{10}$ sold has a poor absorption rate. In my practice, I recently found a form that absorbs five times more than the previous form I recommended, and suggest that patients take 200 to 400 mg daily, with food.

- **Lycopene.** This natural red pigment is found in tomatoes and other red fruits. Lycopene is a powerful suppressor of the initiation process of cancer. I recommend taking 20 to 40 mg daily, with food.

- **Vitamins B$_{12}$ and B$_6$.** In a study of more than 32,000 women, who were followed up for seven years, women who ranked in the highest percentile of blood B$_6$ levels, experienced a 30 percent decrease in incidence of breast cancer, and those who ranked in the highest percentile of blood B_{12} levels experienced a 64 percent decrease. Evaluating your vitamin B_{12} status is important, in order to keep yourself at the highest levels of the normal range. I recommend 150 to 300 mg of B_6 daily, with food, and 5 mg of the sublingual methylated form of vitamin B_{12}, also taken daily, with food. Vitamin B_6 should never be taken without also supplementing B complex; I recommend supplementing 50 to 100 mg of B complex daily, with food.

Activity Maintenance Pillar

- **Physical activity.** Strenuous recreational activities of more than six hours per week decreases the lifetime risk of invasive breast cancer by 23 percent.

  Higher recreational physical activity may also reduce the risk of breast cancer in postmenopausal women. This risk reduction was observed to be more significant with estrogen-positive progesterone-negative breast cancer, a less frequent, but *far* more aggressive and harder-to-treat form of breast cancer. In the beginning of this section on breast cancer, I discussed that this type of cancer is more frequent in women who take selective serotonin reuptake inhibitor (SSRI) medications. It is especially advisable for women in this group to consistently exercise, which, in addition to protecting them from an increase in this specific type of breast cancer, will also help alleviate their depression.

- **Not wearing bras.** The breast has a delicate lymphatic system intended to drain toxins and other substances from the breast. This draining mechanism begins at the nipple, radiates out to drain the perimeter, and finally exits at the underarm.

  Thermography, an alternative method to mammography that I *do not* endorse as a substitute to mammogram, identifies heat in the breast with an increased incidence of precancer or cancer in breast tissue. When breast tissue is examined with thermography immediately after the removal of a bra, the entire breast appears hot. The theory is that the restraining mechanism of a bra cuts off lymphatic drainage and contributes to the development of breast cancer. Although it was not specified, these studies are likely more relevant to the use of underwire bras. Studies have confirmed this.

In 1978, a physician from UCLA Medical Center correlated bra use with elevated breast temperature and an increased risk of developing breast cancer. Since then, numerous studies from the most well-respected medical centers in the world have confirmed the finding that wearing a bra increases your risk of developing breast cancer. In 1991, a Harvard University study and corroborating studies evidenced that women who wear bras increased their incidence of breast cancer 63 percent. A two-year study of 4,700 American women, described in *Dressed to Kill: The Link Between Breast Cancer and Bras* (ISCD Press, 2005), found that the longer a woman wears her bra, the higher her risk for breast cancer. When the authors compared nonusers to women who wear bras eighteen to twenty-four hours a day, the incidence of breast cancer increased by a whopping hundredfold.

My clinical experience shows that within two to six weeks of my patients not wearing a bra, or their switching to an unstructured strapless bandeau bra or other top that does not put pressure on the chest wall as a bra does, many of them enjoy a significant decrease in pain and cysts associated with the development of breast cancer.

As a male gynecologist, I may be speaking a bit out of turn on this issue, and, indeed, I admit that I have not managed to convince my own wife to take a break from her bra. Despite this, I encourage you to consider this compelling medical data and make your own decisions accordingly.

Free of Breast Cancer but Sagging?

Most women are reluctant to forgo bra use because they have been told that doing so results in future sagging of the breast. A Japanese study on the subject concluded that a bra can actually increase breast sagging. Interestingly, this effect was most noticeable in women with larger breasts. It is also my clinical observation that tight-fitting bras, such as those with underwire, cut off the muscle contraction that holds up the breast. Additionally, I have observed that women who wear bras are more likely to slouch, rather than sit or stand erect, failing to contract this muscle.

- **Stop using underarm deodorants.** Women need to sweat. The sweating process drains unwanted substances from the breast region. There is a disproportionately higher incidence of breast cancer in the upper, outer quadrant of the breast, the area closest to the underarm because nearly everything you apply to this area contains toxic substances. Parabens, a cosmetic preservative commonly used in deodorants and other toiletries, has been identified in breast cancer tissue. Aluminum, which is used in antiperspirants, is a toxic material associated with DNA alteration.

  Studies indicate that the longer you use anything on your underarm—antiperspirants, natural or unnatural deodorants, perfumes or colognes, or shaving cream—the earlier your breast cancer diagnosis.

  In my practice, I have long recommended that patients refrain from using any products that contain aluminum or preservatives, or anything that restrains free underarm drainage in any way.

  As an alternative, I suggest applying scented products, like perfume, to the sides of the upper torso or the underside of the biceps, so long as these substances do not come in contact with the sensitive underarm area.

- **Pregnancy.** In adult women, each full-term pregnancy decreases the incidence of breast cancer by 7 percent, and each year of breastfeeding decreases the incidence of the disease by 4.3 percent.

  Women with breast cancer who become pregnant after completing their treatment have a 98 percent survival rate, as compared to the 80 percent survival rate of women who do not get pregnant. In presenting these statistics I want to be clear that I do not condemn any woman for choosing to express her womanhood without having children, by choice or otherwise. What I do want to establish is that the dramatic surge in bioidentical hormones during pregnancy is one of the reasons for these women's decreased risk.

  This benefit is more pronounced in young women. Teenage pregnancy is associated with a decreased risk in developing breast cancer throughout their lives. While I'm not promoting that teenagers become pregnant, the mere fact that they have an increase in estrogen levels at a young age is nonetheless telling. These data are supported by studies on mice in puberty that were given high doses of bioidentical estrogen and progesterone at the time their breasts were developing. The mice had a 60 percent reduction in breast cancer rates and the most aggressive form of breast cancer, HER–2/neu (HER–2), was nearly eliminated in them.

- **Breastfeeding and other nipple stimulation.** Most breast cancer starts in the milk ducts. Studies indicate that each year of breastfeeding decreases the incidence of breast cancer by 4.3 percent. Scientists believe that the nipple stimulation associated with breastfeeding, and any breast stimulation that mimics breastfeeding, releases free radicals from the breast duct and prevents duct obstruction. This is the likely reason for the decrease in breast cancer cases associated with nursing.

  If you don't or choose not to breastfeed, consider making efforts to replicate this nipple stimulation manually. I recommend taking a few minutes two or three times a day—in the shower or when you get into bed at night—to use your fingers to stimulate your nipples in a way that mimics the suckling action of breastfeeding. This is most effective between days fifteen to twenty-eight of your cycle, when progesterone is produced by your body. Progesterone increases the production of oxytocin, a hormone that enhances muscle contraction around the milk duct.

- **Breast massage.** There is no scientific study I know of that established the benefit of breast massage. Yet it seems logical that lymphatic stimulation would be helpful to breast drainage. I recommend your placing your hands flat on your breast, and lightly dragging your fingers from the nipple toward your underarms a few times a day. Visit www .bodymechanics.net to learn more about breast massage techniques.

Hormone Balance Pillar

In my practice, I recommend that my patients optimize their levels of the following breast cancer–fighting hormones:

- **DHEA.** This hormone is one of three androgens that protect women from breast cancer. DHEA suppresses and prevents the growth of the metabolite of estrogen called 4-hydroxy estrone that, when unbalanced, can initiate and stimulate breast cancer (page 147). Supplementing DHEA is highly individualized. For more information on how to use this hormone, see the discussion on DHEA and breast cancer in Chapter 7.

- **Testosterone.** Like DHEA, this second androgen may also be supplemented as part of your breast cancer protection program. Supplementing testosterone is highly individualized. For more information, see the discussion on testosterone and breast cancer in Chapter 9.

- **Dihydrotestosterone (DHT).** This third androgen is a metabolite of testosterone that inhibits the growth of breast cancer.

- **Insulin-like growth factor binding protein-3 (IGFBP-3).** This protein also inhibits the growth of breast cancer cells.

- **Adiponectin.** One of the far-reaching benefits of this hormone, found in fat tissue, is that it arrests angiogenesis, the process by which tumors build new blood vessels in order to progress and spread. The three hormones that promote adiponectin levels are DHEA, HGH, and estradiol.

- **Melatonin.** Our understanding of the importance of melatonin as a general cancer protector is growing. Melatonin decreases cancer cell growth and increases the survival rates of animals with untreated breast cancer. It causes the regression of breast cancer by behaving as an aromatase inhibitor, blocking the cause of breast cancer—where testosterone converts to estrogen in breast tissue, causing the level of estrogen in the breast to be disproportionate to the level in the rest of the body.

  For more information on supplementing melatonin, see the discussion on melatonin in Chapter 14.

- **Progesterone.** As discussed, progesterone provides significant protection from breast cancer. No study that has created concern about the link between hormone therapy and breast cancer used bioidentical progesterone. In the subsection that follows, you'll find a discussion of two major studies where bioidentical progesterone was used as part of hormonal treatment. In both of these studies, the women who used bioidentical progesterone enjoyed a lower incidence of breast cancer than the women who chose to take no hormones (page 349).

  Supplementing progesterone is highly individualized. For more information, see the discussion on progesterone and breast cancer in Chapter 5. For more information on the safety of progesterone, see the discussion of bioidentical progesterone and Provera in Chapter 3.

- **Estriol.** As discussed, in breast tissue estriol attaches to estrogen receptor beta, a process that protects you from cancer. Just as progesterone insures that estradiol uses its strength to benefit the breast, estriol does its part to balance estradiol, as well.

  Additionally, the mere presence of higher levels of estriol has been shown to reduce the risk of breast cancer. In the 1970s and 1980s, estriol served as a marker for high-risk pregnancies. Scientists funded by the U.S. Army Medical Research and Material Command studied the relationship between estriol levels in pregnancy and then followed up the women tested for more than thirty years to determine whether there is the correlation between estriol levels in pregnancy and the future risk of breast cancer. The study concluded that higher estriol levels in pregnancy translated into a 58 percent reduction in future incidence of breast cancer.

  Unfortunately, to date, this naturally protective essential component has never been included in any study of bioidentical and nonbioidentical hormones.

  I regularly recommend supplementing estriol to balance the benefits of estradiol and also to protect my patients from breast cancer. Supplementing estriol is highly individualized. For more information on how to incorporate this powerful tool in your breast cancer prevention program, see the discussion of estriol and breast cancer in Chapter 4.

- **Estradiol.** Am I crazy to suggest that the culprit—estradiol—can protect you from breast cancer? No, I'm not. I will explain, step by step, how bioidentical estradiol together with progesterone, estriol, and all of the other hormones discussed participate in the process of protecting women from breast cancer. No study has ever shown that bioidentical estradiol and bioidentical progesterone hormonal replacement therapy have ever caused an increased incidence of illness or death from breast cancer.

In the only human studies to use bioidentical estradiol and progesterone together, discussed in the subsection that follows, researchers found that this combination promotes a mild to significant decrease in breast cancer.

In another study, women with breast cancer who were given estrogen enjoyed higher survival rates than those who used no hormone treatment, bioidentical or otherwise.

In fact, physicians have found that women who schedule their breast cancer surgeries during the time in their monthly cycle when their estradiol levels are high enjoy better outcomes than women who undergo surgery during a time when their estradiol levels are lower.

To further understand the power of estradiol and estrogen in general, consider the following:

- Estrogen increases apatosis, a mechanism that is protective against cancer and breast cancer.
- Estradiol decreases the ability of breast cancer tumors to resist treatment and improves women's overall outcome, by decreasing interleukin-6, a substance that promotes the growth of cancer tumors, and NFkB, a factor that makes breast cancer resistant to treatment.
- Breast cancer that is estrogen-receptor positive (ER+) is significantly less aggressive and is known to produce significantly better survival rates.
- Estradiol binds to estrogen receptor beta, a process known to decrease proliferation of breast cells and that should have a protective effect against breast cancer.

The specific use of estrogen in breast cancer treatment. Not long ago, before estradiol was vilified as the cause of breast cancer, estrogen(s) were acceptable and successful treatments for breast cancer. Today, we are in an antiestrogen era, so the breast cancer treatment of choice is antiestrogen, as well. Interestingly, when this conventional treatment protocol fails to help patients or stops working after a time, medicine nonetheless turns to estrogen by adding estrogen to a woman's treatment. Once estrogen is added, the conventional treatment begins working again.

Moving beyond "dish medicine." While it is true that when scientists at Northwestern University added estradiol to a dish of breast cancer cells, the cells grew. As discussed at the start of this chapter, a woman's body is far more sophisticated than a dish. When the cancer cells from this dish were implanted in the bodies of a variety of animals, and these animals were supplemented with estradiol, there was a notable reduction in tumor size. This study was repeated several times, and always yielded the same results. Each time, estradiol profoundly reduced the size of the tumors.

Most recently, in 2007, the University of California, Berkeley, and Baylor College of Medicine cooperated on a study (published in *Breast Cancer Research*) in which scientists created an animal model that mimicked the essential elements of human breast cancer. In this study, estradiol treatment decreased the incidence of breast cancer by 67 percent and decreased the ability of breast cancer to multiply by 91 percent.

THE STUDIES: CLEARING THE CONFUSION ONCE AND FOR ALL

Dr. Trudy Bush, adjunct professor of epidemiology and of gynecology and obstetrics at Johns Hopkins, who also held a post in the department of epidemiology and preventive medicine at the University of Maryland School of Medicine, summarized twenty-five years and a whopping fifty reports on HRT and estrogen replacement therapy (ERT), a year before the publication of the Women's Health Initiative (WHI) study. The data from this far more comprehensive report has probably never reached you. Dr. Bush's study concluded: "The evidence did not support the hypothesis that estrogen use increases the risk of breast cancer."

How can one study, a year later, convince scientists to ignore all the far more comprehensive data that came before it? This is particularly striking, considering that the Women's Health Initiative study used neither estradiol, estriol, nor progesterone.

If you look more closely at the studies reported by Dr. Bush, most show a decreased incidence of breast cancer, some show no difference, and a few show an increase of incidence. Yet, all of the studies summarized by Dr. Bush reported a decreased incidence of death from breast cancer. How can this be explained? This is because even the use of estrogen in general provides protection from breast cancer–related death.

Shortly after Dr. Bush's study was published, another study confirmed the reduction of death from breast cancer in women who use HRT, as compared with nonusers.

STUDIES ON USING ESTROGEN ALONE

In studies conducted in the United States, the majority used a chemical estrogen substitute called Premarin. The estrogen-only arm of the WHI study also used Premarin as its form of estrogen. This study showed a 23 percent decrease in the incidence of breast cancer in the first five years of estrogen-only use. Are you surprised to read this? You should be; this important aspect of the WHI study was somehow overlooked in popular reports that created so much fear.

In the first fifteen years of a Harvard University study that followed up more than 28,000 women who used Premarin alone, researchers observed no increase in incidence of breast cancer. Despite these findings, the use of estrogen alone—bioidentical or otherwise—is *not* safe in the long run. Indeed, in this same Harvard University study and others, after twenty years of Premarin-only use, authors observed a 42 percent increase in incidence of breast cancer. Estrogen should never be used alone. It must be paired with bioidentical progesterone and estriol, as it currently is in your body, in order to keep you safe from breast cancer.

In fact, this increase in incidence of breast cancer associated with estrogen-only use is equal to or greater than the risks associated with the lifestyle changes described at the start of this chapter. Specifically:

The increased risk associated with estrogen-only use is equal to the increased breast cancer risk of consuming red meat five times a week— 40 percent.

The increased risk associated with estrogen-only use is equal to the increased breast cancer risk of taking more than fifty days' worth of antibiotics in your lifetime—45 percent.

The increased risk associated with estrogen-only use is a *lower* risk than the increased breast cancer risk of gaining more than thirty-eight pounds in pregnancy—48 percent.

STUDIES ON HRT IN WOMEN WITH BREAST CANCER

In reviewing studies on the most vulnerable group in the hormone debate— women with breast cancer—the data becomes more compelling. Women with a family history of breast cancer who used hormone replacement therapy enjoyed a decrease in the incidence of death from breast cancer.

If you compare the outcome of women with breast cancer who used HRT prior to their diagnoses of cancer, as compared to nonusers prior to cancer, the users enjoy better survival rates and a decreased incidence of cancer metastasis.

Dr. Philip Disaia, a gynecological cancer specialist at the University of California, Irvine, treated women with breast cancer using Premarin and Provera. In comparison to nonuser breast cancer patients, those breast cancer patients who used Premarin and Provera enjoyed an 88 percent survival rate, while nonusers only 63 percent.

In a study conducted at the renowned M. D. Anderson Cancer Center, the group of women with breast cancer who were treated with estrogen enjoyed higher survival rates.

Additionally, a recent Swedish study on cancer recurrence compared women with breast cancer who used estrogen to those who did not, and found that using estrogen did not increase the recurrence of breast cancer.

Finally, two other U.S. studies conducted on breast cancer survivors, published since the Women's Health Initiative study, confirm the safety of hormonal replacement in breast cancer survivors. The first study followed these survivors for more than thirty-two years, and indicates no increase in incidence of death or recurrence of breast cancer. The second prospectively compared two groups of women with breast cancer—one group taking Premarin and a second group that did not. The group assigned to take Premarin included more women with the higher-risk, more aggressive form of breast cancer (estrogen-negative tumors). The study found that the group treated with Premarin had half the deaths and half the metastases of the nontreatment group.

STUDIES USING BIOIDENTICAL HORMONES

Two recent studies from France reviewed the use of bioidentical hormones, including bioidentical estradiol and progesterone (no study has used estriol to date), and the incidence of breast cancer. In one of these studies, more than 54,000 women were studied in three groups. The first group used estrogen and synthetic progestin, and experienced a 40 percent increased incidence of breast cancer, as compared to the third, nonuser group. The second group that used bioidentical estradiol and bioidentical progesterone enjoyed a 10 percent reduction in the incidence of breast cancer, as compared to the third, nonuser group. In other words, women who use bioidentical hormones have lower incidence of breast cancer than those who use none, whereas women who use non-bioidentical hormones have a much *higher* incidence of breast cancer.

The second French study compared users of bioidentical estradiol and bioidentical progesterone with nonusers. More than 80 percent of the women in the user group applied estradiol in the preferred method, directly onto the skin. The nonuser group was characterized by a number of factors that put these women slightly more at risk for developing breast cancer. In the user group, thirty-four out of 3,380 developed breast cancer. In the nonuser group, 205 out of 3,301 women developed breast cancer—a *six-fold increase* in incidence in breast cancer in the nonuser group, as compared to the user group. Note that these favorable results were reported, even though the user group did not utilize estriol, the second important balancing mechanism of estradiol.

Arguably the most well-known authority in the formal study of HRT, Dr. Leon Speroff, professor of obstetrics and gynecology and reproductive endocrinology at Oregon Health & Science University, has publicly spoken at length about the problems associated with the Women's Health Initiative study, including detailing "diagnostic and selection biases, high drop-in and drop-out rates, poorly represented media reports, sound-bite interpretations by 'experts,' epidemiologists giving clinical advice, and the writing of position papers by various medical organizations that, in his opinion, 'were profoundly influenced by medical-legal fears,'" and has announced that Speroff believes that treatment with estrogen and progesterone may actually be beneficial to lowering breast cancer rates when used early in menopause.

THE END OF CONFUSION, THE BEGINNING OF SOLUTION

In a recent article, the authors reported a 7 percent decrease in the incidence of breast cancer after WHI study warnings became public. This decrease was attributed to the success of the WHI study in convincing women to stop taking estrogen. My position is that this statistic is actually based on the decrease in sales of a product that combines Premarin and Provera, warned to be toxic. But that's only one part of the story: the other part is that, since WHI, women have returned to hormone treatments, but this time have chosen risk-free, side effect–free bioidentical hormones.

In my practice, I see women from all over the country and, in some cases, from other nations in the world. Within this patient population, 30 percent of those who used bioidentical estrogen and progesterone prior to the WHI study stopped using these hormones once they heard reports about the study's conclusions. Since then, more than 95 percent of them have restarted their bioidentical hormone treatment.

As discussed in Chapter 3, after the Women's Health Initiative study, women using all manner of hormone replacement therapy were faced with two options: suffering the consequences of living with no symptom relief, or relying on multiple prescription medications to manage the various manifestations of hormone deficiency, including sleep medications, antianxiety medications, antidepressant medications, and a variety of stimulants intended to regain lost memory and cognitive function. Not surprisingly, women quickly found that neither of these options was acceptable to them, as each failed to fully address the conditions for which it was being taken and because each brought on a full spectrum of significant side effects.

Consequently, the majority of these women began using bioidentical hormones. Since then, the number of compounding pharmacies has mushroomed, and most physicians in the part of the state in which I live are effectively forced by their own patients to provide prescriptions for bioidentical hormones to be filled by these compounding pharmacies. As I described, women themselves were leading the grassroots revolution to redefine the standard of care for hormone deficiency. I urge you to do the same regarding your breast cancer concerns. If you believe your family or personal history puts you at risk, don't lose another day to fear. Arm yourself with the science and suggestions provided in this section in order to reduce your risk of developing breast cancer every day.

NOTES

The pages that follow list only those studies actually referred to in this book—a small fraction of the studies and reports used to compile the information presented. For a complete listing of references organized by corresponding chapter and page number, including new resources and studies made available after the publication of this book, consult the "References" section of my website, www.UzziReissMD.com.

Chapter 1

p. 21 **Medical studies proving that eating less increases lifespan:** *Microsc Res Tech.* 2002 Nov 15; 59(4):335–38. Lane, M. A., et al.

p. 22 **50 percent calorie reduction by obese women improves word recall:** *Int J Obes Relat Metab Disord.* 1997 Jan; 21(1):14–21. Kretsch, M. J., et al.

p. 22 **Calorie reduction improves Alzheimer's:** *Interdiscip Top Gerontol.* 2007; 35:159–75. Pasinetti, G. M., et al.

p. 24 **Calorie reduction maintains reproductive hormones and menstrual cycles:** *Exp Gerontol.* 2003 Jan–Feb; 38(1–2):35–46. Mattison, J. A., et al.

p. 25 **Calorie reduction reduces age-related melatonin decline:** *J Clin Endocrinol Metab.* 2001 Jul; 86(7):3292–95. Roth, G. S. *Exp Gerontol.* 2003 Jan–Feb; 38(1–2):35–46. Mattison, J. A., et al.

p. 26 **Studies on caloric reduction in primates:** *Microsc Res Tech.* 2002 Nov 15; 59(4):335–38. Lane, M. A., et al.

p. 26 **Benefits of reducing calories every other day:** *Med Hypotheses.* 2006; 67(2):209–11. Johnson, J. B., et al.

Chapter 2

p. 51 **Exercise decreases IVF outcome:** *Obstet Gynecol.* 2006 Oct; 108(4): 938–45. Morris, S. N., et al.

p. 58 **Higher estrogen levels increase men's attraction:** *Proc Biol Sci.* 2006 Jan 22; 273(1583):135–40. Smith, M. J., et al.

Chapter 3

p. 68 **"The negative impact of the Women's Health Initiative":** *Ob Gyn News.* 2006 Oct 1. Dixon, B. K.

Chapter 4

p. 79 **Levels of estrogen in dairy products are very high:** *J Agric Food Chem.* 2006 Dec 27; 54(26):9785–91. Malekinejad, H., et al.

p. 84 **Estrogen level is associated with aortic calcification:** *NEJM.* 2007 Jun; 316:2591–602. Manson, J. A., et al.

p. 84 **Estradiol (E2) prevents thickening of heart walls:** *Nucl Recept Signal.* 2006; 4:e013. Kim, J. K., et al.

p. 84 **Estradiol (E2) prevents heart failure:** *Basic Res Cardiol.* 2006 Jul 4; Beer, S., et al.

p. 84 **Estradiol (E2) prevents arterial sclerosis:** *J Clin Endocrinol Metab.* 2006 Dec; 91(12):4995–5001. Seli, E., et al.

p. 85 **WHI study and failure to distinguish between bioidentical and chemicalized estrogens:** *JAMA.* 2002; 288:321–33. Women's Health Initiative (WHI Study).

p. 87 **Bioidentical estradiol (E2) cream versus capsules, in weight management and insulin sensitivity:** *Fertil Steril.* 2006 Dec; 86(6): 1669. Micheline, C. C., et al.

p. 87 **Estrogen behaves like an antioxidant:** *Swiss Med Wkly.* 2006 Aug 5; 136(31–32):510–14. Delibasi, T., et al.

p. 87 **Estradiol (E2) decreases IL-6:** *Ginecol Obstet Méx.* 2006 Mar; 74(3):133–38. Saucedo García, R., et al. *J Huazhong Univ Sci Tech Med Sci.* 2006; 26(1):53–58. Wang, Y., et al.

p. 87 **Estradiol (E2) decreases NF-κB:** *Cytokine.* 2005 Aug 21; 31(4):251–57. Liu, H., et al. *J Huazhong Univ Sci Tech Med Sci.* 2006; 26(1):53–58. Wang, Y., et al.

p. 88 **Hypothesis regarding low estrogen levels and permanent memory loss:** *J Neuroendocrinol.* 2007 Feb; 19(2):77–81. Sherwin, B. B.

p. 93 **Migraines increase with changing levels of estrogen:** *Neurology.* 2006 Sept 13. Macgregor, E. A., et al.

p. 94   **"Menstrual migraines":** *Neurology.* 1991 Jun; 41(6):786–93. Silberstein, S. D., et al.

p. 97   **UCLA study on bioidentical estriol (E1) in the treatment of MS:** *Neurology.* 1999 Apr 12; 52(6):1230–38. Kim, S., et al. *J Immunol.* 2003 Dec 1; 171(11):6267–74. Soldan, S. S., et al. *Ann Neurol.* 2002 Oct; 52(4):421–28. Sicotte, N. L., et al.

p. 105   **Estradiol (E2) patch delivers unpredictable amounts of hormone to the bloodstream:** *Fert & Steril.* 2003 Mar; 79(3):534–42. Kraemer, G. R., et al.

p. 107   **Intermittent dosing impairs cognition:** *Brain Res.* 2006 Oct 18; 1115(1):135–47. Gresack, J. E., et al.

p. 108   **Birth control pills and decline in cognition:** *J Nerv Ment Dis.* 1999 May; 187(5):275–80. Rubino-Watkins, M. F., et al.

Chapter 5

p. 113   **Cancer biomarkers increased in group taking Provera, but not in group taking progesterone:** *Breast Cancer Res Treat.* 2007 Jan; 101(2):125–34. Wood, C. E., et al.

p. 113   **Women operated on to remove breast cancer, and progesterone and higher survival rates:** *The Breast J.* 2006 Nov; 12(6):518–25. Kontos, M., et al.

p. 114   **Johns Hopkins study on mortality, cancer, breast cancer, and progesterone:** *Am J Epidemiol.* 1981; 114(2):209–17. Cowan, L. D., et al.

p. 114   **French study evidencing progesterone reducing breast cancer, not progestin:** *Int J Cancer.* 2005 Apr 10; 114(3):448–54. Fournier, A.

p. 114   **French study on how progesterone decreases breast cancer:** *Gynecol Endocrinol.* 2006 Aug; 22(8):423–31. Espie, M., et al.

p. 123   **Progesterone and allopregnenolone levels are lower in PMS:** *Obstet Gynecol.* 1997 Nov: 90(5):709–14. Rapkin, A. J. *Eur J Endocrinol.* 2000 Mar; 142(3):269–73. Monteleone, P., et al.

p. 124   **Bioidentical estrogen to treat PMS:** *Br J Obstet Gynaecol.* 1995 Jun; 102(6):475–84. Smith, R. N., et al.

p. 125   **Absorbable magnesium to treat PMS symptoms:** *Obstet Gynecol.* 1991 Aug; 78(2):177–81. Facchinetti, F. *Clin Drug Investig.* 2007; 27(1):51–58. Quaranta, S., et al.

p. 126   **Physical activity to relieve discomforts of PMS:** *Women's Health.* 2004; 39(3):35–44. Lustyk, M. K., et al.

Chapter 6

p. 132 **HGH improves amylin levels:** *J Cell Biology.* 2004 Feb; 16(4):509–14. Dacquin, R., et al.

p. 133 **HGH treatment improves bone density in hips:** *J Endocrinol Invest.* 2005; 28(8 Suppl):32–36. Agnusdei, D. *Curr Pharm Des.* 2002; 8(23): 2023–32. Svensson, J., et al.

p. 133 **HGH treatment improves growth of bone in the spine:** *Curr Pharm Des.* 2002; 8(23):2023–32. Svensson, J., et al.

p. 134 **Women with low HGH levels do not sleep well:** *Neuro Endocrinol.* 1990 Jan; 5(1):82–84. Astrom, C.

p. 136 **HGH participates in ovarian follicle development:** *Eur J Endocrinol.* 1996 Feb; 134(2):190–96. Bergh, C.

p. 137 **Burn victims have a lower mortality rate when treated with HGH:** *Zhonghua Shao Shang Za Zhi.* 2005 Oct; 21(5):347–49. Chen, G. X., et al.

p. 140 **HGH shown to support and reinforce immune system:** *J Clin Endocrinol Metab.* 1997 Nov; 82(11):3590–96. Khorram, O., et al.

p. 141 **HGH decreases stomach cancer in mice:** *World J Gastroenterol.* 2006 Jun 28; 12(24):3810–13. Liang, D. M., et al.

p. 141 **HGH does not promote cancer in adults or in children:** *Clin Endocrinol* (Oxf). 2006 Feb; 64(2):115–21. Jenkins, P. J., et al. *J Clinic Endo & Metab.* 2001; 86(5):1868–71. Statement, Growth Hormone Research Society.

p. 142 **HGH treatment improves obese diabetic patients:** *Clin Endocrinol* (Oxf). 2006 Apr; 64(4):444–49. Ahn, C. W., et al.

Chapter 7

p. 147 **Supplementing DHEA decreases breast cancer:** *Endo Reviews.* 2003 Apr; 24(2):152–82. Labrie, F., et al. *World J Surg.* 2007 May; 31(5):1041–46. Hardin, C., et al.

p. 147 **DHEA suppressed growth and spread of human breast cancer cells:** *Asia Pac J Clinic Nutr.* 2001; 10(2):165–71. Suzuki, M., et al. *Cancer J.* 2006 Mar–Apr; 12(2):160–65. Gayosso, V., et al. *Breast Cancer Res.* 2005; 76:1132–40. Shilkaitis, A., et al.

p. 147 **Aromatase inhibitors without androgens not as efficient in breast cancer treatment:** *Endocrin-Related Cancer.* 2006 Aug 1; 13:335–55. Labrie, F. *Cancer Res.* 2006 Aug 1; 66(15):7775–82. Macedo, L. F., et al.

p. 148   **General anticancer effects of DHEA:** *Int J Cancer.* 2003 Jun;
105(3):321–25. Ciolino, H., et al. *Cancer Lett.* 1997 Jun 3; 116(1):61–69.
Wang, T. T., et al.

p. 148   **Animal studies on anticancerous effects of DHEA:** *Surgery.*
1997; 121(4):392–97. Melvin, W. S., et al. *Carcinogenesis.* 1984; 5(1):
57–62. Nyce, J. W., et al. *Cancer Res.* 1999 Jul 1; 59(13):3084–89.
Rao, K. V., et al.

p. 148   **DHEA high in POS patients and in young women as
cardioprotective response:** *Eur J Endocrinol.* 2006 Jun; 154(6):883–90.
Dagre, A., et al.

p. 149   **DHEA increases pancreatic cells:** *Febs Lett.* 2006 Jan 9; 580(1):285–
90. Medina, M. C., et al.

p. 151   **DHEA improves muscle mass and strength after resistance exercises:**
Am J Physiol Endocrinol Metab. 2006 Nov; 291(5):E1003–8. Villareal,
D. T., et al.

p. 151   **DHEA reverses age-related changes in fat mass:** *Clin Endocrinol* (Oxf).
2000 Nov; 53(5):561–68. Villareal, D. T., et al. *Eur J Endocrinol.* 2006 Oct;
155(4):593–600. Hernandez-Morante, J. J., et al.

p. 152   **DHEA improves bone density:** *J Clin Endocrinol Metab.* 2006 Aug;
91(8):2986–93. Jankowski, C. M., et al. *Cell Mol Immunol.* 2006 Feb;
13(1):41–45. Wang, Y. D., et al.

p. 152   **DHEA megadose produces increased sex drive and better orgasmic
response:** *J Women's Health Gend Based Med.* 2002 Mar; 11(2):155–62.
Hackbert, L., et al.

p. 155   **Caloric reduction decreases age-related drop in DHEA levels:** *Exp
Gerontol.* 2003 Jan–Feb; 38(1–2):35–46. Mattison, J. A., et al.

p. 155   **Lower levels of DHEA associated with increased mortality:** *Ann
Epidemiol.* 2006 Jul; 16(7):510–15. Glei, D. A., et al.

p. 157   **Higher levels of DHEA as response to polycystic ovarian syndrome:**
Eur J Endocrinol. 2006 Jun; 154(6):883–90. Dagre, A., et al.

p. 158   **Misleading test results:** *J Clin Endocrinol Metab.* 1994 Jun;
78(6):1360–67. Morales, A. J., et al.

p. 158   **DHEA reduces proliferation of liver cancer:** *Int J Oncol.* 2004 Oct;
25(4):1021–30. Mayer, D., et al.

p. 159   **Misleading test conditions in dosing mice with DHEA:** *Cancer Lett.*
1997 Dec 23; 121(2):125–31. Metzger, C., et al.

Chapter 8

p. 171 **Pregnenolone decreases cholesterol levels in complete hormonal replacement programs:** *Med Hypotheses* 2000 Dec; 59(6):751–56. Dzugan, S. A., et al. *Gastroenterology.* 1984 Aug; 87(2):284–92. Turley, S. D., et al.

Chapter 9

p. 182 **Testosterone significantly reduced women's fear response:** *Biol Psychiatry.* 2006 May 1; 59(9):872–74. Hermans, E. J., et al.

p. 183 **Testosterone supplementation has positive effect on depression:** *Climacterk.* 2004 Dec; 7(4):338–46. Studd, J., et al.

p. 190 **Premarin known to increase level of sex-binding globulin:** *Gynecol Endocrinol.* 1993 Dec; 7(4):251–58. Compagnoli, C., et al.

p. 190 **Women lose sexual drive and function when taking Prozac:** *J Affect Disorder.* 1998 Mar; 48(2–3):157–61. Seidman S. N., et al.

p. 191 **Misunderstanding regarding definition of female sexual deficiency:** *J Clin Psychology.* 2005 Nov; 66(11):1409–14. Nelson, J. C., et al. *J Sex Med.* 2005 May; 2(3):291–300. Basson, R., et al.

p. 192 **Genital arousal peaks for hours after application of testosterone cream:** *J Sex Med.* 2006 May; 3(3):541–49. Apperloo, M., et al.

p. 196 **Caffeine reduces hair loss associated with testosterone:** *Int J Dermatol.* 2007 Jan; 46(1):27–35. Fischer, T. W., et al.

Chapter 12

p. 244 **Zoloft ineffective at elevating mood:** *JAMA.* 2002 Apr 10; 287(14):1807–14. Hypericum Study Group.

p. 244 **Saint-John's-wort more effective than Prozac:** *J Clin Psychopharmacol.* 2005 Oct; 25(5):441–47. Fava, M., et al.

Chapter 14

p. 276 **Abnormal sleep patterns correlate to lower life expectancy:** *Am J Manag Care.* 2006 May; 12(8 Supp):5214–20. Doghramji, K., et al.

p. 280   **Estrogen and progesterone first defense against insomnia:** *J Br Menopause Soc.* 2004 Dec; 10(4):145–50. Polo-Kantola, P., et al.

p. 286   **Melatonin helps adjust to a new time zone:** *J Mol Microbiol Biotechnol.* 2002 Sep; 4(5): 463–66. Parry, B. L. *Cochrane Database Syst Rev.* 2002; (2): CD001520. Herxheimer, A., et al.

Chapter 15

p. 296   **Fruit consumption does not benefit memory:** *Neurology.* 2006 Oct 24; 67(8):1370–76. Morris, M. C., et al.

p. 298   **Animals and BDNF:** *Neuroscience.* 2002; 112(4):803–14. Molteni, R., et al.

p. 298   **Consuming saturated and trans fats lowers cognitive function:** *Neurology.* 2004 May 11; 62(9):1573–79. Morris, M. C., et al.

p. 298   **Doesn't take long for unfavorable fats to have negative effect on cognitive function:** *J Nutr Health Aging.* 2006 Sep–Oct; 10(5):386–99. Bourre, J. M.

p. 301   **Zinc improves spatial working memory and visual memory:** *Br J Nutr.* 2006 Oct; 96(4):752–60. Maylor, E. A., et al.

p. 308   **Hydergine improves memory loss:** *Acta Pharmacol Sin.* 2006 Jan; 27(1):1–26. Wang, R., et al. *Curr Med Res Opin.* 1986; 10(4):256–79. Huber, F., et al. *Arch Neurol.* 1994 Aug; 51(8):787–98. Schneider, L. S., et al.

p. 310   **Suboptimal thyroid levels can be seen on MRI/CT scans:** *Neuroepidemiology.* 2006; 27(2):89–95. Reitz, C., et al.

p. 311   **Testosterone improves women's visual and spatial memory:** *Psychoneuroendocrinology.* 2004 Jun; 29(5):612–17. Aleman, A., et al.

p. 312   **HGH improves memory loss:** *Horm Res.* 2005; 64 Suppl 3: 109–14. Van Dam, P. S. *Horm Res.* 2005; 64 Suppl 3:100–108. Maruff, P., et al.

p. 314   **Treadmill running improves brain cell production in hippocampus:** *Brain Res.* 2006 Aug 9; 1104(1):64–72. Ledo, M., et al.

p. 314   **Study on improved cognitive performance in women ages 59 to 68:** *J Physiol Pharmacol.* 2006 Sep; 57 Suppl 4:417–24. Zlomanczuk, P., et al.

p. 315   **Interpersonal stress in adults enhances memory failure:** *Psychol Aging.* 2006 Jun; 21(2):424–29. Neupert, S. D., et al.

p. 316   **Yoga, prayer, tai chi, and meditation have healing effects on the brain:** *Psychol Rep.* 1997 Oct; 81(2):555–61. Naveen, K. V., et al. *Percept Mot Skills.* 1999 Jun; 88(3 pt):765–70. Fabbro, F., et al. *Arch Phys Med Rehabil.*

2001 Sep; 82(9):1283–85. Shapira, M. Y., et al. *Int J Clin Exp Hypn.* 2004
Oct; 52(4):434–55. Wagstaff, G. F., et al.

p. 316   **Sleep deprivation is a chronic stress inducer:** *Metabolism.* 2006 Oct;
55(10 Supp 2):20–23. McEwen, B. C.

p. 318   **UCLA study on short-term lifestyle changes that significantly
improve memory:** *Am J Geriatr Psychiatry.* 2006 Jun; 14(6):538–45.
Small, G. W., et al.

Chapter 17

p. 326   **Women's fears of breast cancer far exceed reality:** Presentation South
Atlantic Association Ob/Gyn, Boca Raton. 2004. Levin.

p. 328   **Increased risk of breast cancer from oral contraception when taken
between ages fifteen and twenty:** *Eur J Cancer.* 2005; 41(15):2312–20.
Jernstrom, H., et al.

p. 330   **Studies demonstrating association between iodine deficiency and
breast cancer:** *Trans NY Acad Science.* 1970; 32:911–47. Eskin, B. A. *Breast.*
2001 Oct; 10(5):379–82. Venturi, S. *J Mammry Gland Biol Neoplasia.* 2005
Apr; 10(2):189–96. Aceves, C., et al.

p. 332   **CLA inhibits cell proliferation in cancer cells:** *Exp Mol Pathol.* 2005
Oct; 79(2):118–25. Albright, C. D., et al.

p. 332   **Whey and whey acid proteins inhibit proliferation and spread of
breast cancer:** *Cancer Lett.* 2007 Jan 8; 252(1):65–74. Nukumi, N., et al.

p. 333   **Grape juice, grape seeds, and red wine serve as aromatase inhibitors in
breast cancer prevention:** *Ann NY Acad Sci.* 2002; 963:229–38. Chen, S.
Cancer Res. 2006 Jun 1; 66(11):5960–67. Kijima, I., et al. *Breast Cancer Res Treat.*
2001 May; 67(2):133–46. Eng, E. T., et al. *Ann NY Acad Sci.* 2002 Jun;
963:239–46. Eng, E.T., et al.

p. 333   **Resveratrol prevents breast cancer:** *Mol Nutr Food Res.* 2005 May;
49(5):452–61. Ulrich, S., et al.

p. 335   **Fiber and decrease of breast cancer in perimenopausal women:** *Int J
Epidemiol* 2007 April; 36(2):431–38. Cade, J. E., et al.

p. 335   **Indole-3-carbinol increased 2-hydroxy estrone:** *J Cell Biochem Suppl.*
1997; 28–29:111–16. Wong, G. Y., et al.

p. 335   **Indole-3-carbinol reduces epidermal growth factor receptors:**
Apoptosis. 2006 May; 11(5):799–812. Moiseeva, E. P., et al. *Carcinogenesis.*
2007 Feb; 28(2):435–45. Moiseeva, E. P., et al.

p. 337   **Vitamins B$_{12}$ and B$_6$ decrease incidence of breast cancer:** *J Natl Cancer Inst.* 2003 Mar 5; 95(5):373–80. Zhang, S. M., et al.

p. 339   **Bra use increases breast temperature:** *Lancet.* 1978 Nov 4; 101. John, M.

p. 339   **Use of bras increases incidence of breast cancer:** *Eur J Cancer.* 1991; 27:131–35. Hsieh, C., et al.

p. 339   **Bra use for eighteen to twenty-four hours a day increases breast cancer risk more than 100-fold:** *Dressed to Kill.* 1995. Avery Singer, S., et al.

p. 340   **Bra use increases breast sagging:** *J Hum Ergol.* 1990 Jun; 19(1):53–62. Ashizawa, K., et al.

p. 340   **Use of products on underarm increases breast cancer:** *Eur J Cancer Prev.* 2003 Dec; 12(6):479–85. McGrath, K. G.

p. 341   **Mice studies with high doses of estrogen and progesterone show a decrease of breast cancer growth and spread:** *Breast Cancer Res.* 2007 Jan 26; 9(1):R12. Rajkumar, L., et al.

p. 341   **Breastfeeding decreases incidence of breast cancer:** *Lancet.* 2002; 360(9328):187–95. Sitieri, P. K., et al.

p. 344   **Higher estriol levels in pregnancy reduce future breast cancer:** Prospective study of risk of breast cancer with estrogen during pregnancy; unpublished studies, Public Health Institute, Oakland, funded by U.S. Army Medical Research. DAMD 17-99-1-9358 et al.

p. 345   **Bioidentical estradiol (E2) and progesterone decrease breast cancer:** *Int J Cancer.* 2005 Apr 10; 114(3):448–54. Fournier, A., et al. *Gynecol Endocrinol.* 2006 Aug; 22(8):423–31. Espie, M., et al.

p. 345   **Women with breast cancer given estrogen enjoyed higher survival rates:** *J Clin Oncol.* 1999 May; 17(5):1482–87. Vassilopoulou-Sellin, R., et al. *Menopause.* 2003 Aug; 10(4):277–85. Decker, D. A., et al.

p. 346   **Estradiol (E2) treatment decreases breast cancer and its ability to multiply:** *Breast Cancer Res.* 2007 Jan 26. Lakshmanaswamy, R., et al.

p. 346   **Dr. Bush's report on the safety of HRT and ERT:** *Obstet & Gynecol.* 2001 Sep; 98(3):498–508. Bush, T. L., et al.

p. 347   **Reduction of cancer death with use of HRT:** *Am J Obstet Gyn.* 2002; 186:325–34. Nanda, K., et al.

p. 347   **WHI study on Premarin use and decreased breast cancer:** *JAMA.* 2002 Jul 17; 288(3):321–33. Rossouw, J. E., et al.

p. 347   **Fifteen-year Harvard University study on estrogen use with no breast cancer:** *Arch Intern Med.* 2006 May; 166(9):1027–32. Chen, W. Y., et al.

p. 347   **Twenty-year Harvard University study:** *Lancet.* 1997; 350(9084): 1047–59.

p. 348   **Family history of breast cancer, and use of HRT:** *Ann Inter Med.* 1997; 127(11):75–78. Sellers, T. A., et al.

p. 348   **Use of HRT prior to breast cancer diagnosis improves survival rates:** *Br J Cancer.* 1999 Jul; 80(9):1453–58. Jernstrom, H., et al. *Am J Obstet & Gynecol.* 2007 Apr; 196(4):342.e1–9. Schuetz, F., et al.

p. 348   **Premarin and Provera improve survival rates in breast cancer treatment:** *Women's Health.* 2001 Oct. Disaia, P. J.

p. 348   **M. D. Anderson Cancer Center study on estrogen and decreased breast cancer:** *J Clin Oncol.* 1999 May; 17(5):1482–87. Vassilopoulou-Sellin, R., et al.

p. 349   **Other studies on estrogen and increased survival rates:** *Obstet & Gynecol.* 2001 Sep; 98(3):498–508. Bush, T. L., et al. *Am J Obstet Gyn.* 2002; 186:325–34. Nanda, K., et al.

p. 349   **Estrogen decreases breast cancer recurrence:** *J Natl Cancer Inst.* 2005; 97(7):533–35. Von Schoultz, E., et al.

p. 349   **Additional studies showing increased survival rates with use of estrogen:** *Am J Obstet Gyn.* 2002 Aug; 187(2):289–94. Puthugramam, K., et al. *Menopause.* 2003 Jul–Aug; 10(4):277–85. Decker, D., et al.

p. 349   **Thirty-two-year study showing safety of HRT use in breast cancer survivors:** *Am J Obstet Gyn.* 2002 Aug; 187(2):289–94. Puthugramam, K., et al.

p. 349   **Breast cancer survivors receiving estrogen treatment show decreased mortality and recurrence:** *Menopause.* 2003 Jul–Aug; 10(4):277–85. Decker, D., et al.

p. 349   **Bioidentical estradiol (E2) and progesterone reduce mortality rates in breast cancer, when compared with non-use:** *Int J Cancer.* 2005 Apr 10; 114(3):448–54. Fournier, A., et al.

p. 349   **French study of bioidentical estradiol (E2) and progesterone shows reduced mortality rates, when compared with non-use:** *Gynecol Endocrinol.* 2006 Aug; 22(8):423–31. Espie, M., et al.

p. 350   **"Diagnostic and selection biases . . .":** *Ob Gyn News.* 2006 Oct 1. Dixon, B. K.

p. 350   **WHI study warnings:** *Ob Gyn News.* 2007 Jan 1; 42(1):1. Jancin, B., et al.

RESOURCES

WHERE TO BUY NATURAL SUPPLEMENTS

The nutritional supplements recommended in this book are available at health food stores and over the Internet. Be a savvy consumer of nutritional supplements: Insist on the best-quality products you can find. If a product is not producing the expected results, consider trying another brand—the quality of ingredients used in nutritional supplements varies widely. If you are unable to find products that satisfy your needs, visit my website to find information on obtaining the supplements that I offer to the women who visit my office, and products that my clinical results are based on.

WHERE TO BUY BIOIDENTICAL HORMONES

Compounding pharmacies are the most reliable sources of bioidentical hormones. Conventional pharmacies carry only premanufactured medications, while compounding pharmacies create individualized combinations, doses, and forms of bioidentical hormones, nutritional supplements, and medications for physicians and patients. They use high-quality ingredients and follow government regulations.

Since the publication of my first book on the subject of women's natural hormone balance, a wonderful thing has happened in the world of bioidentical hormone therapy. Women have led a revolution that has caused mainstream healthcare providers—who had never considered recommending natural hormones—to educate themselves about this powerful set of tools. I have always been a great supporter of compounding pharmacies and the health-care professionals who work with them.

Some of the hormones discussed in this book require a prescription from your physician. If your doctor won't provide one, you may want to contact a compounding pharmacy and ask for the names of health professionals in your area who use natural hormones (medical doctors, osteopathic doctors, and in some states naturopaths and nurse practitioners). I train physicians individually about the methodology of my hormone treatment protocols. At the time of this writing, my physician recommendations include:

Joseph McWherter, M.D.,
and Associates
Toll-free: 888-FEM-CNTR
(336-2687)

The FEM Centre–Fort Worth
709 West Leuda St.
Fort Worth, TX 76104
Telephone: 817-926-2511
Fax: 817-924-0167

The FEM Centre–Colleyville
6221 Colleyville Boulevard, Suite 150
Colleyville, TX 76034
Telephone: 817-251-6533
Fax: 817-251-0340

Daniela Paunesky, M.D.
Allyn A. Brizel, M.D.

Renaissance Medical Center
3400 Old Milton Parkway
Building C, Suite 380
Alpharetta, GA 30005
Telephone: 770-777-7707
Fax: 770-777-7789

I currently work with and am personally involved in the development of the hormone compounds of this compounding pharmacy:

Pharmix Center
Toll-free: 866-421-5722
2560 East Sunset Road
Suite 120
Las Vegas, NV 89120

Telephone: 702-541-6023
Fax: 702-405-8135
E-mail: info@pharmixcenter.com
URL: www.PharmixCenter.com

As with nutritional supplements, the quality of ingredients in biodentical hormones and in the mediums used in the creams, gels, drops, pills, or capsules that carry them, is extremely important as far as absorption levels and results. The products of this pharmacy are the same products that my clinical results are based on. If you have any special concerns, sensitivities, or allergies, you should speak directly to the pharmacist.

INDEX